FAST YOUR WAY TO HEALTH

FAST YOUR WAY TO HEALTH

J. HAROLD SMITH

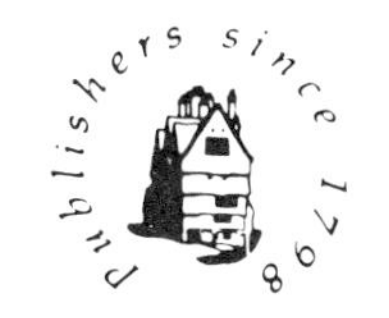

THOMAS NELSON PUBLISHERS
Nashville • Camden • New York

Published in Nashville, Tennessee, by Thomas Nelson, Inc.

Printed in the United States of America.

All Scripture quotations are from the King James Version of the Bible unless otherwise indicated.

Tenth printing

RADIO BIBLE HOUR, INC.
P.O. Box 99
Newport, Tennessee 37821

Library of Congress Cataloging in Publication Data

Smith, J Harold, 1910-
Fast your way to health.

Bibliography: p. 122
1. Fasting. I. Title.
RM226.S54 613.2 79–1437
ISBN 0-8407-5676-3

CONTENTS

FAST YOUR WAY TO HEALTH

Introduction

Fasting has been around for a long time. In more recent years, however, there has been more talk about it by health enthusiasts in particular. The Christian world has been less quick to respond to the new emphasis on the fasting phenomenon. This is rather surprising considering that fasting as a practice to deepen one's relationship to God is deeply rooted in Bible history. On the other hand, as this book points out, the reluctance of many Christians to fast can be traced to the abuses of the practice through the centuries by the early church and some ascetics. Then there are those Christians who have been practicing periodic fasting for a long time in private and have discovered it to be a channel of power and true spirituality. Some of God's choicest saints through the ages have fasted.

This book is an effort to call attention to a practice that I have personally found to be of great benefit but which is being neglected or overlooked by much of the world today. It is a subject that is close to my heart. I feel qualified to write about it not only on the basis of my education, but more importantly, because the Bible teaches it, and I have practiced fasting on a number of occasions. I know the physical, mental, and spiritual benefits that will accrue to the individual who fasts periodically. I can commend the practice to you.

As a young man my greatest desire was to become a doctor of medicine. I longed to relieve suffering humanity.

As a result of this intense desire, I spent eight years in the study of chemistry, anatomy, biology, and medicine, all the scientific studies that would lead me to be a doctor of medicine. I graduated from Furman University, Greenville, South Carolina, on August 28, 1932, fully intending to spend the rest of my life in the field of medicine. But God had other ideas. On September 4, 1932, exactly seven days after receiving my degree, I had a born-again experience that changed the direction of my life. I did not go into the practice of medicine; instead, I felt God's call to become a minister of the gospel of Christ. Thirteen days later, on September 17, 1932, I preached my first sermon and have averaged speaking four times each day since.

The need for men of medicine cannot be denied; I would be among the first to laud them. But as a medical doctor, I could only give men temporary relief from their sickness; now through Christ, I preach an eternal relief from the sickness of sin. In medicine all patients sooner or later die; but in Christ they can live forever.

The fact that you have picked up this book may mean that you have a weight problem. If so, it is safe to assume you aren't exactly proud of those extra ugly pounds. You are probably more than a little tired of your second (and third) chin. You sense it when people laugh at your bulges, and the general feeling of despair is a heavy additional weight you could do without. You'd like to gain the victory over your fat problem. Then, this book will be worth its weight in "fat" for you.

Not only will you lose pounds if you do as this book suggests, but on the basis of personal experience and the example of others, I can assure you that you will not only feel better physically, but mentally as well. The rejuvenation will be three-fold in physical, mental, and spiritual benefits.

Fasting is the oldest known method of weight control; moreover, it has a biblical basis. *Nothing in this book should be considered as medical advice or regarded as medical treatment,* but fasting, as a means of losing weight and cleansing the system of toxins to improve one's health, is becoming recognized in more medical circles. *It is important, however, if you are going on an extended fast that you have the approval and guidance of your physician.*

Fasting, when done correctly, can be a tremendous experience. You are about to launch on a journey that will have surprises at every turn of the road. In particular, I commend the practice of periodic fasting as a means of spiritual discipline, i.e., a turning of one's back on food as you confront the far greater need to satisfy the cravings of the inner man in giving yourself to God in worship and praise. That is true biblical fasting.

Fasting for health reasons has its place and this is not to be minimized; but let the reader be cautioned in advance that wrongly motivated fasting is worse than no fasting, and the Bible gives strong warnings about it.

This book attempts to cover the three-fold aspects of fasting: physical, mental, and spiritual. I am especially interested in seeing the reader grasp the importance of the right combination of the three, with special emphasis on the biblical meaning of the fast.

1

The Key to a Healthier, Longer, and More Satisfying Life

If someone told you they *knew* what could be done to make old age wait and to slow down the aging process, you'd no doubt be quick to pump them for information. Who really wants to grow old? Oh, we want to live to a ripe old age, but we don't like the idea of the discomforts, the physical limitations, the possibility of senility, and other characteristics of old age. What are the main causes of disease and aging? Why can't you look at sixty as you looked at thirty? Is there actually something one can do to stave off body deterioration? What contributes to a body growing old?

Strength Depends on the Weakest Vital Link

Medical science teaches that the main cause of disease and aging is to be found in biochemical suffocation, that is the systemic disorder that interferes with normal processes of cell metabolism and cell regeneration. More simply put it means that there is a process going on in our bodies continuously whereby assimilated food is built up and then broken down to be used by our bodies with an accompanying release of energy for all vital life processes. If we are slowing down that process by an accumulation of waste products in our tissues, it stands to reason that there will be an interference with the nourishment and oxygenation of cells.

You are therefore as healthy and as young as your

smallest links, the cells. The question is how can you keep those cells in peak condition? What can you do so your cells don't degenerate and break down?

Fast To Restore Health

I have been fasting since I was age forty. It is as beneficial now as when I went on my first extended fast of twelve days.

I am not exaggerating when I say that I believe I would be dead now if I had not learned this great method of cleansing my body of its filth. This method traces its roots to the Bible and the medical lore of other eras when great men of medicine prescribed fasting. In more recent years, research studies, particularly in Europe, have demonstrated that fasting is a safe measure and has beneficial healing and restorative effects.

Interestingly enough, although our ancestors didn't have access to research studies and modern medicine's findings, they often by necessity had to live on very little if any food. Yet such people in many instances lived long lives. Look at the heroes and heroines of the Bible and trace their long life spans. Have you ever wondered why they lived so long? Obviously they did something right. We know they ate far differently than modern man does today, and fasting was commonly practiced. This ought to say something to us.

Periodic abstinence from food had beneficial effects on primitive peoples' health as their bodies used these times to cleanse themselves of toxic wastes. During such times digestive and eliminative organs were given a rest, and there was a restoration and normalizing process taking place whereby the glands and vital organs were stimulated to rebuild new cells.

To develop a mind that will enable you to consider fasting, I want you to think of your body as being a refinery.

When a fast begins and the body stops taking in food, the blood and energies that have been occupied in digestion, assimilation, and elimination disengage themselves and direct their attention elsewhere. The entire body turns into a "refinery."

The blood, which acts as the sewer system of the body, flows throughout the body in this process of refinement. Each day of the fast, the blood, the body, the mind, and the soul get cleaner and cleaner. The cleansing realities of fasting and the beneficial effects of such a thorough cleansing cannot be disputed, as future chapters will reveal.

Someone has suggested that fasting is like turning off the motor of your car and coasting downhill. I like that. Think about it. There is not one cell in our bodies that is not helped by giving it an opportunity to rest and be cleansed. In a normal healthy body, about half of one's cells are in peak working condition; one fourth are usually in the process of growth, and the other fourth in the process of dying and replacement.[1] It's these dying cells that cause aging and other health problems. Because of nutritional deficiences, sluggish metabolism, sedentary life, and overeating with accompanying digestion problems, our cells are unable to resist disease—and there are the accompanying ills and symptoms of advancing age. Where there is quick and effective elimination of dead and dying cells, there is the building and growth of new cells. Fasting promotes the process of such elimination, and in that process the body rids itself of toxic substances that are interfering with the nourishment and oxygenation of the cells, the building blocks of our bodies.

Your Building Blocks

When we talk about building blocks, we aren't talking about toys! Actually, your body is composed of billions of tiny cells. While the biblical psalmist didn't use the word "cell," he did talk about the complexity of the body's refinery:

For thou hast possessed my reins: thou hast covered me in my mother's womb. I will praise thee; for I am fearfully and wonderfully made: marvellous are thy works; and that my soul knoweth right well. My substance was not hid from thee, when I was made in secret, and curiously wrought in the lowest parts of the earth. Thine eyes did see my substance, yet being unperfect; and in thy book all my members were written, which in continuance were fashioned, when as yet there was none of them (Ps. 139:13–16).

These tiny building blocks need all the help they can get. What are you doing to help? Have you ever tried fasting?

Have You Ever Wondered About Wrinkles?

Wrinkles and "crow's feet"—who wants them? Who needs them prematurely? Sometimes they appear long before chronological age indicates that this is normal and to be expected. Cell replacement has been impaired by what you are doing to your "refinery." Doesn't it stand to reason if you give that refinery an opportunity to slough off its refuse that something is bound to happen? It is a known physiological fact that during a fast, even though no nourishment is being supplied to the body, there is a building up of new, healthy cells.

As the diseased and dead tissues decompose and burn, a transformation takes place in those "delicate, inner parts" of our bodies. We are cooperating with God in tissue repair. What does this mean?

The first time a friend heard me say "less chance of crow's feet" she was elated. The first recognition that age is creeping up on you is disconcerting to say the least. When you realize that your profile isn't quite what it used to be, you begin to wonder what you can do to slow the aging process. Fasting will help.

Cooperating With the Creator

There is an old German proverb that states: "The illness that cannot be cured by fasting, cannot be cured by anything else." I agree just about one hundred percent with this proverb. Fasting permits the healing functions that God has built into our bodies to work. We call it nature, but it is actually the Creator's divine laws of healing at work in our bodies.

Why have we, such an enlightened race, been so long in discovering this marvelous, God-given way of cooperating with our Creator in the maintenance of health? Could it be that our known enemy, Satan, has blinded us to the great biblical doctrine of fasting?

Mental and Spiritual Rewards

I have already indicated that fasting has its roots in the Bible. The Bible teaches fasting. Fasting pleases God. More than one Bible personality found it difficult to come into God's presence on a full stomach! Self-indulgence through overeating or failure to discipline one's self to a God-honoring fast is a strong indicator that the natural or carnal instincts are in control.

Not only does the discipline of fasting reap physical rewards, but mental and spiritual rewards are every bit as great, if not greater. Authentic biblical fasting was always a spiritual exercise.

God's Servants Fast

Fasting as taught in the Bible is a much-neglected teaching both in and out of the church. An in-depth study of the subject, however, reveals that the early church and the saints of old fasted frequently, and the hand of God moved in surprising and often miraculous ways on their behalf. It is an exciting study and one I will pursue in subsequent chapters.

A look at the spiritual lethargy, coldness, and deadness that characterizes much of the church today causes the concerned individual to ask "Why?" and "What can be done?" I am personally of the opinion that, among other things, a return to the biblical teaching of fasting would bring a renewed vigor to churches throughout our land.

The Bible promises that fasting, when approached as a spiritual exercise with a calling upon God for the will to begin and the strength to endure, will release God's power according to His promise. In particular, that promise is recorded in Isaiah 58:8.

> Then shall thy light break forth as the morning, and thine health shall spring forth speedily: and thy righteousness shall go before thee; the glory of the Lord shall be thy rereward.

Here we see a three-fold promise: *Light breaking forth,* which speaks to me of a mental equipping where fresh light from God's Word and God Himself (as we reach out to Him in more consecrated prayer and specific thought) comes in a powerful way. We live in what the Bible calls "a darkened world," and light is surely required if we are to do God's work in God's way. Second, there is *the promise of health* that I have briefly outlined in previous paragraphs and which will be treated more fully in subsequent chapters. And finally, *the promise of righteousness* and all this implies. In the Bible, fasting was always considered a channel of power. If one's spirituality and power and gifts of the Spirit were to be operative, then this need for the righteousness that comes from above was clearly evident. This the Bible faithfully records, and biblical characters sought it through prayer and fasting. It was an age-old prescription taught by God as revealed through His prophets and men of old.

There are eighty-six references in the Word of God that speak on fasting. This neglect today of a subject that has such obvious results both for the physical and spiritual well-being of an individual is difficult to explain. As with other biblical teachings of great value that have been overlooked or given little attention, man is the lesser and, one might add, the loser.

Perhaps we have avoided fasting because it has connotations of fanaticism. One thinks immediately of India's Mahatma Ghandi, the political statesman the Christian world may have regarded more as a mystic than a hero. Or one thinks of entertainer Dick Gregory who made headlines with his fasts; or novelist Upton Sinclair who stumbled upon the benefits of fasting largely by accident.

Modern man, unaccustomed for the most part to sacrifice and not too willing to submit himself to rigorous self-control and stern discipline, backs off from those subjects and teachings that might infringe too much on that from which he derives so much pleasure—eating. And so we Americans are the best-fed nation on the face of the earth, yet researchers increasingly are pointing out that our diets are dangerously deficient in the nutrients essential to good health, and that we have an alarming health situation in the United States. To suggest to the millions of overweight and otherwise unhealthy people in this nation that fasting is a regimen to help them lose weight and regain health is to open one's self to censure, criticism, and skepticism. Yet, that is precisely what this book is all about; moreover, and what is of greater importance, it can be shown that fasting is a spiritual exercise, the benefits of which will produce fruitful living and a new dimension of growth in the inner man that is more satisfying than gorging one's self with food.

Fasting Benefits All

Obese people may only be interested in the physical benefits of fasting, philosophers only in the mental benefits, and religious people in the spiritual benefits. But fasting has benefits for all; and all can benefit in a three-dimensional way.

2

My Own Experience with Fasting

What qualifies me to write on the subject of fasting? I've done it! Not once, nor twice, but often. These fasts have been of varying duration, but each has yielded rich physical, mental, and spiritual benefits.

With my medical education background I felt competent to practice fasting on these numerous occasions. Fasting is, however, something that many medical doctors do not recommend. You have no doubt heard the statement, "Just what the doctor ordered." Fasting is not generally just what the doctor is going to order.

Actually, throughout medical history fasting has been recognized as the oldest, most dependable therapeutic curative method known to man. Early man may well have learned this from animals. You don't see dogs, cats or other animals eating when they are sick. Hippocrates, Galen, Paracelsus, and many other "greats" of medicine prescribed fasting.[1]

What these ancient men of medicine knew, and what many medical doctors and others have discovered, is that fasting itself is not a *cure* in the modern meaning of that much abused term, but fasting is a period of physiological rest. This rest provides an opportunity for the body to do for itself what it cannot do when it is busy refining or processing food. But in our drug-oriented culture we have departed from that which was instituted by God Himself for both physical and spiritual benefits. It is granted, of course, that fasting must be undertaken by those who are prepared to sensibly follow certain precautions.

Dr. Paavo Airola, world-famous nutritionist, naturopathic physician, and award-winning health writer, writes convincingly of the scientific studies being made around the world (particularly in Europe) which show the prophylactic, therapeutic, and rejuvenative effects of fasting. Such studies done in Sweden, Germany, Russia, England, and elsewhere prove that controlled fasting leaves the participants stronger and with more vigor and vitality. Dr. Airola particularly recommends juice fasting and explains that in Europe this is practiced on a grand scale.[2]

Water Fasting

I have had the most success with water fasting. On one of these water-only fasts, which I refer to as an "absolute fast," I lost forty-four pounds in twenty-eight days.

On February 12, 1976, I ate dinner. I did not take into my body anything but water after that until Friday morning, March 12, 1976. This fast lasted four full weeks.

During those twenty-eight days, I carried on all of my work as usual. I preached sixty-one times and traveled over seven thousand miles. I dictated letters, prepared material for our magazine, and performed all the responsibilities that are mine as president of our radio broadcast. There was time and energy to work in my flower and vegetable garden, and I even went fishing!

But how did I feel? That question is asked with regularity when the subject of fasting comes up. The idea seems to be that you have to eat something every day if you are going to "feel good." One woman seriously stated, "But you have to keep something in your stomach at all times or it will grow together." Let us lay that and other old wives' tales to rest right now.

There are those who actually believe a person will die if no food is taken into the body for ten days. Others think you will lose your mind and "go crazy" without food. Secular and biblical history—and current literature—have much to teach us about such fallacies.

How did I feel? Every fiber of my sixty-five-year-old body *rejoiced*! I felt great! Yes, it's true there were times when, if I suddenly stood up, I would feel light-headed. But the dizziness was only momentary.

There were several times, especially after a long day of mental exertion, when I felt tired, but every day I was getting nearer my goal. My mind became as clear as a spring of pure mountain water. I had a feeling of cleanness of mind, body, and soul. It was an invigorating sort of feeling. I felt drawn closer to God. Not only was I feeling better physically, but I knew my mental faculties were sharper and with that came an increased spiritual awareness. God assured me of the answer to certain prayers and burdens that were on my heart when I began the fast.

I have been on only one fast longer than this one. It too was a water-only fast, but it lasted forty days.

I had always felt that I would never have the power with God in preaching, in understanding the Bible, and in helping people that I needed until I had read the sixty-six books of the Bible while on an absolute fast. During that forty-day fast, I read the entire Bible once and half of it a second time. I preached eighty-two times, traveled over ten thousand miles, and carried on my duties as president of the Radio Bible Hour broadcast.

I kept a chart on the twenty-eight-day fast. As you will note, the chart reveals that when I began the fast I weighed 218 pounds. This was a good deal more than I had ever weighed before. I am six feet tall.

DATE	WEIGHT	ACTIVITIES
2/13	218 pounds	Preached eight times. All duties.
2/14	215 pounds	Worked in yard and garden. Fished.
2/15	213 pounds	Attended church. Rested.
2/16	211 pounds	Preached eight times. All duties.
2/17	209 pounds	Preached six times. All duties.
2/18	205 pounds	Preached twelve times. All duties.
2/19	202 pounds	Preached twelve times. All duties.
2/20	198 pounds	Preached twelve times. All duties.
2/21	197 pounds	Outing with family.
2/22	196 pounds	Attended church. Rested.
2/23	195 pounds	Began revival.
2/24	193 pounds	Revival. Spoke twice each day.
2/25	190 pounds	Revival. Spoke twice each day.
2/26	189 pounds	Revival. Spoke twice each day.
2/27	188 pounds	Closed revival.
2/28	186 pounds	Continued regular schedule.
2/29	186 pounds	Continued regular schedule.
3/ 1	184 pounds	Continued regular schedule.
3/ 2	184 pounds	Continued regular schedule.
3/ 3	182 pounds	Continued regular schedule.
3/ 4	181 pounds	Continued regular schedule.
3/ 5	181 pounds	Continued regular schedule.
3/ 6	179 pounds	Continued regular schedule.
3/ 7	178 pounds	Continued regular schedule.
3/ 8	178 pounds	Continued regular schedule.
3/ 9	176 pounds	Continued regular schedule.
3/10	175 pounds	Continued regular schedule.
3/11	174 pounds	Continued regular schedule.

My family and the staff of the Radio Bible Hour can testify to the truth of my forty-four-pound weight loss.

Ignoring the Wrong Kind of Advice

During this fast I had to learn to ignore the "advice" of well-meaning friends. I heard such things as "Preacher, you look starved!" I looked at myself, and I really didn't look at all like the gaunt-faced children in magazine advertisements seeking donations for underfed orphans.

Nor did I bear any resemblance to the emaciated victims of famine countries.

Another said, "Aren't you weak? Will you make it through the day?" Would I make it through the day? Even midway through the fast, at 189 pounds, it was obvious I wasn't suffering.

Others said, "Please drink some juice."

"This peanut brittle candy sure is good, preacher!"

"Have a hot dog."

"Surely you could suck on a popcicle."

"These French fries are out of this world!" After one look at the protruding stomach hanging over "Mr. French Fry's" belt, I wanted to tell him he'd be out of this world sooner than his allotted time if he didn't shape up.

One fellow said, "Man, you are going to kill yourself. You will come down sick." Every day I was getting farther and farther away from a sick bed or a hospital stay. The Bible talks of our health as springing forth speedily when we fast (Isa. 58:8). I knew the Word of God was not a lie. I knew my friends meant well, but I was determined with God's help not to be deterred in this quest for better health, mental peace, and spiritual enrichment. I did not want to be among those digging their own graves with their forks, knives, and spoons. To those who expressed their fear of fasting, I expressed my own belief that fasting is not nearly so deadly as *feasting*.

Benjamin Franklin once said, "I saw few die of hunger, but of eating, over a hundred thousand." It was he who was fond of quoting, "God heals and the doctor takes the fee."

The Talmud declares, "In eating, a third of the stomach should be filled with food, a third with drink, and the other third left empty."

We do not look to the wisdom of the sages of the past often enough. There was a time in my life when I shared the views expressed by well-meaning friends. But then I was unlearned and ignorant of the facts because I had not bothered to inform myself. I, too, thought that an absolute fast for twenty-one days, twenty-eight days, or forty days was an impossibility; and if someone did it, surely he would be endangering his health. Then, at age forty, I began researching the subject. I am in much better health today than when I reached mid-life.

The Reins of Health

I believe that we hold the reins of health in our own hands. Though we cannot expect to remain free from some natural infirmity that all flesh is heir to, I, personally, cannot, at the time of this writing when I am sixty-five, complain of one thing as it pertains to my physical well-being. It is simply miraculous, but I am thankful that God directed me into the great biblical truth of fasting.

The number is uncountable of those whose bodies need a thorough house cleaning. This can best come through fasting. When a person goes into an extended fast, sometimes it seems you are surely going to get sick or die, and the old flesh lets you know it resents going without food. But there is victory ahead if you will not give in to those initial hunger cravings.

What You Can Expect

Hunger!

When I began the twenty-eight-day fast, I was hungry for about the first three or four days. This is a normal reaction to a complete cutoff from food intake. Don't be alarmed by this craving for food. You will find yourself thinking that just one bite won't matter, and who is to know the difference. The answer to that, of course, is that *you* know and God knows. You are only cheating yourself.

How do you *not* yield to temptation? First of all, recognize who the tempter actually is. ". . . Resist the devil, and he will flee from you" (James 4:7).

Karen Wise, who considered herself a fat failure, went from 340 pounds to being the target of "a wolf whistle," as she puts it in her challenging book, *God Knows I Won't Be Fat Again.*[3] But it didn't happen overnight. There were years of conflict, turmoil, and severe temptations to break her diet. But Karen learned to cooperate with God, and four years later she emerged a winner. Today, Karen, who is slim, beautiful, and has a hard-won self-respect that was worth all the effort, would tell you that God still works in the lives of human beings. It begins at that point, however, of doing what the Bible says: "Submit yourself therefore to God . . ." (James 4:7).

Hunger is a normal reaction and not to be considered a bad sign. Other good signs will be a growing acidosis whereby your tongue will become coated with a white covering and your breath will take on the odor of acetone. This is probably one of the more unpleasant side effects of fasting, but about midway through my twenty-eight-day fast, my tongue began to lose its white coating and the odor of acetone began to disappear. But acidosis is a good sign because the body is sloughing off and ridding itself of its toxicity. This represents a cleansing process.

Along with the growing acidosis, I lose my appetite completely. This is another normal and good sign. This indicates that gastric irritation, which produces the sensation of hunger pangs, has ceased.

Dizziness. I soon learned to avoid quick movements. The first time you experience momentary dizziness may come after sitting for awhile or upon suddenly getting out of bed. If you remember not to move too quickly at this point in your fast, you will be able to maintain your balance. There is no danger in this; it is a sure sign the fast is working for you. Fasting lowers the amount of oxygen in the body. Some people experience a state of euphoria, a type of "high." It is similar to the low-oxygen state long-distance runners encounter. Your body and brain are working under a new set of conditions. The brain has switched to a different fuel system and is using ketone bodies to replace the normal supply of glucose. However, the fat that is being expended for ketone body utilization has proved to be a reliable nutrient for the brain.[4]

What is happening is that your body is mobilizing its protein stores and only a relatively small amount of glucose is available. The carbohydrate stores are quickly depleted. This usually happens between the fourth to the thirteenth day and will return to pre-fast levels by the twenty-first to the twenty-sixth day.

You may experience some headaches accompanied by this lightheaded or dizzy feeling, but in the process of burning up stored fats and proteins, the stored poisons in your body are being used up also. This is a good sign.

Dr. Otto Buchinger, M.D., considered by many to be one of the greatest fasting authorities in the world, claims that in fasting our bodies become "refuse disposals," whereby they actually burn the accumulated rubbish material that has accumulated.

Think about that. Wouldn't you like to rid your body of whatever it is that is contributing to fatty deposits, tumors, abcesses, and the general deterioration of your cells? Doesn't it stand to reason that as the old or diseased cells are decomposed a resurgence of a general feeling of well-being will take over your body?

Body odors, bad breath (with an accompanying heavy coating of the tongue), and your mouth feeling as if it were full of cotton—these are good signs, not bad ones, and are well worth enduring for the ultimate benefits that will accrue.

Vacation For Your Digestive System

When you give your digestive system a complete vacation through fasting, you will experience great joy in seeing your fat rolls disappear. That's putting it quite bluntly, but if you are at all overweight, then you know the distress those ugly fat rolls and bulges bring. Parting with these "spare tires" and unsightly lumps and bumps will help you regain self-respect and a new self-image.

The physiological rest that is afforded the digestive and other organs of our bodies during a fast would be reason enough to fast. But, as I have previously indicated, there are mental and (most important) spiritual rewards as well.

After years of practicing and teaching fasting, I am convinced that God uses this means to help many people lose excess weight and relieve suffering from rheumatism, bursitis, stress, skin diseases, allergies, hay fever, asthma, nervous exhaustion, poor circulation, high blood pressure, and kidney and bladder diseases. Recently it has been discovered that fasting has helped provide relief for schizophrenics and others who are mentally disturbed.[5]

After my last twenty-eight-day fast, and following an earlier forty-day fast, my tongue finally cleared up and became as pink and clean as a little baby's. My breath became sweet. I was surprised to see the dead skin come off my feet and blemishes on my body clear up—seemingly miraculously. Everything about fasting for me has been beneficial. But you need to take certain precautions and follow certain rules. This book is meant to help you make discoveries that can provide lifelong benefits.

3

Facing Fears of Fasting

I have many friends who are doctors of medicine and favor fasting. Had it not been for the knowledge and skill of one of these great doctors, I would long ago have been in my grave. Many other doctors, who are also my friends, do not recognize the wisdom of fasting. They, as the patients they care for, have a fear of fasting.

Fasting may not be what doctors universally are ordering, but from the Bible, we have the evidence that God approves of fasting. It's possible that there may be very sound reasons why *you* will *not* be able to undertake a prolonged fast. Sincere doctors do not agree on the advisability of fasting. Some insist that fasting upsets an individual's metabolism and brings other adverse effects. Other doctors disagree and are quick to tell of patients who got rid of painful arthritis as a result of fasting.[1] One individual lost eighty-one pounds and in the process shed an irritable disposition *and* regained his handsome looks. However, only you and *your* doctor can make the determination for yourself.

Fasting is certainly one of the least expensive diet programs ever devised! Ideally, you should be supervised, and logically, short of going to a clinic where experienced supervisors do nothing but monitor fasters, your doctor is the one to act as supervisor. If your doctor declares you to be in satisfactory health and does not favor fasting, you may wish to try and locate a doctor who will agree to supervise. Recognize at the outset that no living thing can go indefinitely without food, but fasting is always safe within the limits of the organism's power of self-help. Dr. Herbert M. Shelton, an expert in the field of therapeutic fasting, cautions that the faster's physical condition should determine the length of a fast. There will always be variables that must be handled and decided upon with common sense. The approach must be flexible, humane, understanding, and wise. This has been emphasized by others and I agree. We are human beings, not machines.

Fear Excess Fat, Not Fasting

There is no reason for you to fear fasting. Fear should grip you, however, if you are carrying around twenty, thirty, fifty or more pounds of extra fat.

Obesity is an ugly sounding word. A woman friend relates that the first time she heard her doctor use the word to describe her overweight condition, which at the time she didn't even feel was "too much overweight," she wanted to crawl under the examining table and hide. "It really shocked me," she said. "I thought the word was meant to describe people *grossly* overweight, but my doctor explained that even ten or fifteen pounds was overweight. Overweight is overweight and the medical term for it is *obesity*."

Let's face it, obesity is a serious health problem, but medical doctors have been sounding warnings for years that most so-called reducing diets are harmful. Many diet methods do help a person to shed pounds, but medical reports show that damaged health may be the result.

I know individuals who have "tried everything" to lose weight without success. It was when they tried fasting and stuck with it for a few days at a time, gradually lengthening the duration of their fasts, that they discovered they had finally found a way to shed pounds. Then when they worked at restructuring their daily intake of food, they cleared the hurdle that spelled victory over their obesity problem.

Danger!

There are dangers lurking in every obese body. When you are from twenty to forty pounds overweight for your age, height, and skeletal structure, then you are skating on thin ice. A check with your insurance agent will confirm that insurance premiums are higher for the grossly obese. One insurance underwriter said privately, "If any group of people is flirting with not being able to purchase life insurance, it is people who are overweight and have a history of obesity. Life insurance premiums are rated according to one's health, past medical records, and the life expectancy of a person according to age. If an individual has lost weight, he still may not qualify for insurance coverage at standard rates if his past records indicate he has had a long problem with obesity. This is not to say this person could not obtain insurance coverage, but he would be rated several different levels beyond standard and the rates would be considerably higher."

This same insurance agent explained that being overweight could totally exclude someone from qualifying for coverage. Blood pressure is watched very closely in life insurance or health insurance applicants. It is recognized that the obese are in greater danger of high blood pressure, strokes, heart failure, poor blood circulation, diabetes, gall bladder trouble, shortness of breath, stomach problems, constipation, burping and indigestion, headaches, fatigue, nervousness, and almost always a shorter life span.

Many obese men are troubled with prostate gland trouble. This trouble can develop into benign or malignant tumors. Overeating contributes to the enlargement of the prostate. Fasting, many times, gives wonderful relief from this urethral obstruction and relieves the retention of urine in the bladder.

It is amazing what an absolute or juice fast will do in reducing inflammation of the colon, more commonly known as colitis. Fasting, as previously emphasized, is surely not a cure-all. When practiced regularly and faithfully, fasting is more a preventative than an agent of healing. Who can deny that preventive medicine is to be preferred! Stay in good health by regular fasts. I am not suggesting twenty-eight day or even ten-day fasts, but periodic short rests for one's stomach and organs. (More on length of fasts in another chapter.)

If fasting were injurious to the body, I do not believe it would be mentioned as much as it is in the Bible. Jesus would never have done anything to injure His body, and we have the biblical record that He fasted forty days! Jesus didn't get hungry until His fast ended; then He hungered and the devil tempted Him to turn stones into bread and eat.

I am of the firm opinion, or I wouldn't be writing this book, that fasting will add years to one's life. And fasting will enable an individual to enjoy the best health ever experienced. But, best of all, I believe that one draws closer to one's Maker in the process.

Some fasting specialists claim that the average individual who eats properly and takes a series of fasts regularly might be able to add from twenty to thirty-five years to his life span. Why die at fifty-five? Why not live to be ninety? Why be guilty of committing a type of "suicide" twenty or more years before our work is done just by failing to fast periodically and eat sensibly and in moderation? The older we become, the greater the need for eating less and fasting. As body activities slow down and we exercise less, the body requires much less food to keep it functioning properly.

Weight Loss and Control

Use your head! Millions of overweight Americans could

have slimmed down a long time ago by doing just that. You can't pick up a magazine without seeing a feature article extolling someone's latest way of losing weight. Dieting has become a national pastime. We know more about counting calories than we do about Christ. People are desperately searching for ways to shed pounds. Ironically, even as they frantically search, they are carrying the perfect weight loss secret right in their own heads. You can lose all the weight you want quickly—and keep it off permanently—through fasting and a program of sane and moderate eating.

How much can you expect to lose? It will vary according to individual body metabolism, but you can expect to lose at least a pound each day. In the back of your head, you may think you'll starve if you miss over six meals or two days without food. Get this lie out of your head. Most people who are twenty-five pounds overweight could go without food for sixty-three meals or twenty-one days. You may rest assured that if you would go on this kind of a twenty-one day absolute water or juice fast, you would lose your extra twenty-five pounds. No fast of this duration should be undertaken, however, unless supervised.

Most overweight people who fast for twenty-one days, it has been shown, do lose twenty-five pounds or more. In addition one who fasts for twenty-eight days may expect an extra eighteen percent weight loss. For example, a man weighing 230 pounds at the start of a twenty-eight day fast, may expect to lose forty-two pounds at the end of twenty-eight days. At the end he should weigh between 185 to 188 pounds. A woman weighing 160 pounds at the beginning of a twenty-eight day fast, should weigh between 125 to 128 pounds. Who wouldn't like to see this happen?

I know many fat people who have given up the idea they will ever lose their extra pounds. They classify themselves as fat failures. Yet they have never tried fasting; or, if they have tried, their will power gave out on them after the first twenty-four hours. Or would it be more accurate to say their "won't power"? I wish there were some magic formula whereby we could all recapture our vanishing will power right at the moment we need it most.

Much is being said and written these days about behavior modification programs to aid overweight people. And such programs can work. But in the final analysis, each of us is still going to be responsible for our behavior, and the worst battles are often fought in regard to food. Just about the time you think you have the battle won, that overwhelming feeling of emptiness hits and you succumb. "Tomorrow I'll do better." "Tomorrow I'll start over." And tomorrow is the day you worried about yesterday.

"I'm starved," you say to yourself. And you listen to your stomach growl its complaint. "I'm ravenously hungry," you complain to your husband, wife, or co-worker. "I can't stand this," and self-discipline flies out the window.

Hunger is a vital bodily function and we need regularly recurring reminders from our stomachs that they need food. So not only is eating a pleasure, but it is a necessity for survival. But the hunger pangs will diminish, and I can tell you from actual experience, after the first few days, they will leave almost entirely. If you can exert that will power and overcome that hurdle, you will be well on your way to total victory. Isn't it worth some added effort? To eat or not to eat is purely personal. Properly motivated fasts, when one seeks the help of the Almighty and is genuinely concerned about total well-being, stand a far better chance of succeeding than an improperly motivated fast for simply selfish reasons.

There is no denying it—going without food is a discipline. Linking it to a purpose, making it a spiritual exercise, is going to make all the difference in the world. Fasting for many is a fast way to weight loss. It also is an invaluable aid to personal sanctity.

4

Me? A Belly Server?

Sometimes the Bible states things so bluntly it's enough to make a person wince! Such a place can be found in Romans 16:17 and 18. ". . . mark them which cause divisions and offenses contrary to the doctrine which ye have learned; and avoid them. For they that are such serve not our Lord Jesus Christ, but their own belly . . ."

Who or What Is Your Master?

The "belly servers" live to satisfy their own lusts. Their own private interests and the indulgence of their earthly appetites consume their thoughts, their time, and a disproportionate amount of their efforts. "Wait, just a moment," you say, "you're coming down awfully hard on overweight people, aren't you?" Let us not make the mistake of assuming that the apostle is here referring only to one's appetite for food. "Lust" could be pride in one's accomplishments, an overambition to succeed, covetousness for luxuries (cars, a fancy home, clothing, entertainment), lascivious living (lust, sensual reading materials)—whatever supplants God in one's mode of living. And yes, *even* Christians are guilty of this. The apostle Paul said it: ". . . whose God *is their* belly . . ." (Phil. 3:19).

But as it relates to the subject of fasting and the consuming passion many people have for overindulgence in food, it can quite literally be stated that they do have a problem with their "bellies." Karen Wise, the girl who succeeded in losing 225 pounds, tells of her remarkable odyssey in which after losing all that weight the skin from her stomach hung down to her thighs. "I had to have it surgically removed. They cut from one hip to the other and took off all the excess skin. I had a flat stomach for the first time in years. When I had been home from the hospital a few days, I noticed that the skin around the incision was beginning to turn black and went back in to have the doctor look at it. My skin had been stretched for so long that it was so unhealthy it didn't have enough life left in it to heal properly.

"I had to go back in again and they did the same thing all over, cutting back further and trying it again with what proved to be better skin. It's still a shock to look at myself and not see a hanging stomach."[1]

Realistically facing the facts, one is confronted with the not-so-glamorous aspect of obesity, and Karen Wise knows whereof she speaks. "Belly servers."

The biblical writer would have us recognize that the gratifying of one's sensual appetite carries with it a price tag. In terms of what it does to our health and chances for longevity, it's a horrendous price to pay. This perversion of one's better judgment and deception of one's own heart is a form of enslavement—not unlike that of the alcoholic or the "smokeaholic."

It has always seemed to me something of an indictment of far too many in the Christian world whose stretched stomachs show an altogether too obvious affection and fondness for food. More of us need to read such books as Dr. Stanley Mooneyham's *What Do You Say To a Hungry World?* (Word Books, 1975). The protruding bones and the pitifully distorted bodies with stomachs stretched out of shape, these—and the haunting looks from the eyes of the victims of starvation—should shame us into changing our ways. We are confronted with immense economic, political, and logistical issues that complicate our response to the needs of a hungry world. Mooneyham wisely stresses that God doesn't expect us to surrender our enjoyment of life for perpetual guilt feelings. "Among the joys, food itself is a celebration," says Mooneyham. But in a reexamining of ourselves, surely there must come the recognition that we can live more sensitively. We have established in this country (and other affluent countries) a cultural pattern of waste. As we gobble up the goodies, let us assess our values. Perhaps we need to pray: "Lord, renew a right spirit within me. Lord, set me free from the power that makes of me a 'belly server.' "

The apostle Paul was on many occasions a weeping preacher not unlike the Old Testament prophets. More than once he said, "To write the same things is safe"; or he would say, "I have told you often, and now tell you even weeping," and he would repeat a warning. So convinced was this great preacher of the need for careful watching of one's appetites (including food) that, in more than one place, he speaks of "belly servers." We sacrifice the favor of God when we make food (or anything else) more important than giving heed to the solemn warnings of the biblical writers.

Habit Hunger

This enslavement to food can be traced in part to what I call being "habit bound." When an excess of carbohydrates, sweets, and starches are eaten, these go into the stomach to contact the gastric juices and other acids within. These soon produce a condition that causes habit hunger. We can become enslaved to these hunger feelings and that's just what they are—feelings. Actually we are not *really* hungry.

Are You a "Foodaholic"?

There are more "foodaholics" in the world today than one would imagine. People in this category are in love with food and have an almost continuous desire to gorge themselves with anything edible. Apply the following test. It may indicate if you qualify as a "foodaholic."

1. Are you the fastest eater in your family?
2. Do you crave food when you are unhappy or disappointed?
3. When eating a buffet dinner, do you worry about how much you have on your plate, compared to the others who are eating?
4. Do you wake up in the middle of the night worrying about your appetite?
5. Are you embarrassed when someone asks you about your eating habits?
6. Do you have to have a little snack just before retiring for bed at night?
7. Do you ever slip into the kitchen at midnight to ease a hunger pang?
8. When you come into the house, is your first stop at the refrigerator?
9. Do you nibble on food while the rest of the family is preparing the meal or waiting for you to finish preparations?
10. Do you eat so much that you feel uncomfortable?

How did you rate on this test?

Whether we want to hear it or not, the Bible is a very practical book when it comes to matters even such as this. Jesus left us the perfect example. Many are astonished when they are told that Jesus said, ". . . Take no thought for your life, what ye shall eat, or what ye shall drink. . . . Is not the life more than meat . . . ?" (Matt. 6:25).

This is taken from the well-known "Sermon on the Mount," in which Jesus gave important teachings on a variety of subjects. The value of these teachings has not diminished with time. In this sermon, more was said of fasting and eating than about alms and prayer. This is worth pondering. Jesus was concerned about the practical aspects of living, such as eating. But there was always a proper balance in Jesus' life, as there should be in ours.

Eating binges are often a cover-up for psychological miseries. The drunkard drinks to drown his problems; the "foodaholic" eats to assuage his needs.

True or False Hunger?

We eat much of the time as a matter of routine. At other times, we eat as a social activity. Still, on other occasions, we eat when there is nothing else to do, and as a momentary distraction, eating is a pastime that relieves some unpleasant worries. Much of the time what we mistake for hunger is gastric irritation. This explains why after three or four days on a fast what we call hunger pangs are considerably lessened.

The gnawing in the stomach, the feeling of weakness, and other seeming manifestations of hunger are thought by many who have researched the subject to be more emotionally-rooted discomforts than actual and true hunger. We are really creatures of habit. Fasters, and I can attest to this myself, will tell you that when your body is signaling you to end a fast, there will be a conscious desire for food, but there is no pain nor irritation. According to Dr. Herbert Shelton, a fasting specialist, "normal hunger is indicated by a general body condition—a universal call for food—which is localized, so far as localization takes place, in the mouth, nose, and throat, just as is the sense of thirst. There are no 'hunger pangs' associated with *genuine* hunger; there is only a pleasant sensation in the nose, mouth and throat and a watering of the mouth."[2]

Dr. Shelton is considered to be a foremost authority on fasting. He has conducted over thirty thousand fasts and supervised both short and long fasts for people of all ages in varying states of health. It is his contention that true hunger is intermittent and will manifest itself when there is a genuine need for food. Shelton says, "It is never continuous; individuals who are 'always hungry' are really displaying pathological symptoms. Am I implying that most people do not really know when they are hungry? I am indeed. Beginning almost with birth and the three-times-a-day stuffing program that is common in our so-called modern civilization, average individuals in average communities never experience genuine hunger."[3]

This doctor believes that true hunger is selective rather than indiscriminate. In contrast to compulsive eaters who are often plagued with longings to eat but never know exactly what they want to eat, the authentically hungry person will not gulp greedily, nor will he demand "luxurious dishes." He tends to be satisfied with plain fare.

One of the distinct advantages of fasting is that you can develop entirely new eating patterns once you do resume eating. For many people this means limiting themselves to smaller portions, or eating one main meal a day. This readjustment in one's thinking and eating is a form of behavior modification that is actually the thing most needed by overeaters and obese people. This has the benefit of helping maintain a long-term weight loss.

Surely one of the important benefits of fasting has to be a recognition that what one calls hunger pangs are not necessarily that at all. Upton Sinclair, a notable faster, described what happened to him when he lost interest in food. "You almost forget that there is such a thing as eating; you can look at food without any more desire for it than you have to swallow marbles and carpet tacks. But then suddenly appetite returns . . . and you find that you can think of nothing but food."[4] This sensation is the body sending out its signal that true hunger exists.

But you question, what about those victims of disasters—those who survive plane crashes, are marooned on islands, and so on—who have even been known to resort to cannibalism. Feelings of desperation will send people into unreasoning acts. Severe anguish and panic force people to do repulsive things. Thinking they are dying of hunger, survivors of disasters do not know they can stay alive without food and that the intense feelings of hunger will subside.

Do Yourself a Big Favor

When I see someone whose belly gives him or her away, I want to gently tap them on the shoulder and say: "You're not doing yourself a favor, you know." Dr. Airola maintains that systematic undereating is the *number one* health and longevity secret. Overeating is one of the main causes of disease and premature aging. Have you ever seen an obese person age one hundred or older? Scientific studies both in this country and elsewhere show that overeating is one of the prime causes of degenerative diseases.

When Will We Learn?

We are so slow to learn. We close our eyes to the truth and block out any information that would interfere with pleasurable habits we've acquired. And eating is pleasurable.

But if we will give up the ostrich-like stance, pull our stubborn necks up out of the proverbial sand, wipe the sand out of our eyes, and give *all* our senses an opportunity to grasp fundamental truths that are so vital to good health and a longer, more satisfying life, we may yet discover that the less we eat, the less hunger we experience, and the better we will look, act, and feel. Besides, who wants to be called "a belly server"?

5

You Are as Old as Your Arteries... and Other Physical Advantages of Fasting

A writer friend says that people are misusing and abusing their bodies and are serving themselves a heaping portion of death.[1]

Americans are spending more than $120 billion annually on health, compared to $39 billion a decade ago. Health care expenditures amount to more than 8 percent of the gross national product. That's an increase of more than one-third from the 6 percent level of ten years ago. Are you aware that the cost of an average hospital stay has increased from $311 in 1965 to more than $1,000 in 1977?[2]

We aren't taking care of our refineries!

Who is to blame? You are individually responsible. And if you are the head of a household, you are responsible for the members of your family.

We hear much about pollution of the atmosphere; it is time we start focusing on self-pollution and rid ourselves of what is contributing to it.

Cholesterol Sludge

In the purification process that takes place during fasting, the toxins are literally flushed out of the body. As unneeded fat is burned up and eliminated, healing occurs in vital organs. There is a saying: *You are as old as your arteries*. Clogged arteries are feared by overweight people and individuals with known heart conditions. Our arteries are soda straw thin. Hardening of the arteries means simply that fatty materials and calcium have accumulated to the point that the artery walls lose their resiliency and actually become hard. Those of us who believe in periodic fasting followed by a change in eating habits feel that this can bring about a change in one's blood pressure and a healing in one's arterial walls.

More and more we are coming to the recognition that many diseases today are due to wrong eating habits, incorrect food combinations, acidulous foods, and our use of commercially prepared foods full of additives. Is it any wonder that our digestive systems react the way they do? How are we going to rid our bodies of these accumulated poisons unless we periodically flush them out through fasting?

I have already assured you that the weakness and dizziness sometimes encountered during a fast is good. This is a sure sign that the refining process is succeeding. As the blood becomes thinner, purer, and more highly refined, it goes through the blood vessels searching out the poisons and impurities. I am convinced that one of the best ways to fight cholesterol, clogged arteries, and high blood pressure is by nature's way: fasting.

God has blessed our arteries with a self-cleaning system. The lifeless matter decomposing in our bodies needs expelling, and the body will burn and digest its own tissues in a process called autolysis, or self-digestion. You rightly question, "Isn't that dangerous?" Dr. Airola emphasizes that the body will not do this indiscriminately. In fasting the body feeds itself on the impure and inferior materials first. The essential tissues, vital organs, glands, nervous system, and brain are not damaged or digested in fasting *when we are doing this on a controlled basis,* i.e., watching our bodily signals (more about this in a later chapter) and ending the fast in a proper way.

The Creator had a plan for man's diet. God made

provision for His created beings so that they could survive. That plan is stated very simply in Genesis 1:29.

> I have given you every herb bearing seed, which is upon the face of all the earth, and every tree, in the which is the fruit of a tree yielding seed; to you it shall be for meat.

Early man grew up in this idyllic state in which he routinely consumed natural, raw, whole fruits, vegetables, and grains. Later, modest amounts of meat were added. But the natural and raw foods contained all the natural vitamins, minerals, and enzymes he needed for optimum health. Modern man has tampered with the Creator's plan—we cook, freeze, preserve, artificially color and contaminate, treat, and denaturalize our foods. We aggravate the malfunctioning of cells and abuse our bodies. We bring about cholesterol sludge and other serious health problems.

Doctors warn that this scummy, lifeless matter may choke arteries, hamper blood flow, and damage the heart. A friend recently shared with me that her brother awakened one morning at 1:30. He complained of chest pain and said he thought he was having a heart attack. When his wife said, "Let me call the doctor," he replied, "Oh, it's probably just gas." He went to the bathroom and a few minutes later returned to bed. He turned out the light, but shortly thereafter his wife sensed something to be wrong. Quickly she turned on the light. Her worst suspicions were soon realized. She couldn't move him. Instantaneous death. The autopsy revealed clogged arteries. How true it is that we are as old as our arteries!

Right now millions of people are suffering from high cholesterol. Unless they take proper actions to clean out their systems, they, too, will one day have clogged arteries. It could be a matter of life or death. Most people are not even aware that this could be happening to them. What a pity! If they only knew what fasting could do for them. It could give them a new lease on life and add years to their lives.

Consider what a small effort this actually is—to discipline one's self periodically to fast to rid one's system of impurities and give one's body a much-needed rest—and what you stand to gain.

As far back as 1950, medical scientists began extensive investigations into the role of foods in cholesterol build-up. Thousands of victims of strokes and heart attacks were diagnosed and interviewed, and the findings were carefully studied. Over eight hundred basic foods were analyzed. Close to five thousand laboratory tests and even autopsies were performed. From this mountain of worldwide research came startling new discoveries.

Scientists know that certain foods containing cholesterol and saturated fats are not necessarily harmful when correctly prepared. But, when processed incorrectly, they become downright dangerous to the body. They know that cholesterol scum can become hardened like chalky soap powder, sticking onto artery walls. With passing time, it may choke the arteries, and the victim will end up with crippling diseases, or worse, in death. Cholesterol has been called "the invisible killer," for good reason.

High blood pressure is known to be second to hardening of the arteries as a cause of heart disease in this country. The arteries narrow, pressure builds up behind constricted vessels, and the work of the heart is increased. This is frequently referred to as hypertension, something that is not limited to the old. Contributing causes are tension, excessive eating, coffee, tea, tobacco, alcohol, too much salt in one's diet, and a general over-taxing of one's nervous system. Treatment is usually directed to depressing the nervous system—drugs are administered, surgical procedures (removal of the thyroid gland and portions of the sympathetic nervous system), elimination of salt, or other suspected causes. But when fasting is tried, there is a marked reduction in blood pressure. Why? Because the toxic load in the system is reduced, the nervous system becomes less irritated, the functions of the kidneys, adrenal, thyroid, and pituitary glands are given an opportunity to return to a more normal state, and the causes that have produced the condition in the first place are eliminated. It is time we cut out causes, not vital organs, as we seek better health.[3]

Away With Myths

Even physicians at one time believed that if one were to go without food for six days, the heart would collapse and death would result. That myth, in fact, persisted until the famous Cork hunger strike in 1920.

Dr. Herbert Shelton tells about this in his book *Fasting Can Save Your Life*. It was the Easter Rebellion of Irish patriots Terence Mac Swiney, the Lord Mayor of Cork, and others who when arrested went without food for periods ranging from seventy to ninety-four days. They demonstrated by their long fasts the fallacy of the "heart collapse from the lack-of-food" theory.

There are plenty of other such instances throughout history—both biblical and secular—that destroy the "heart collapse" myth.[4] The world of science has since abandoned this fallacy.

There is another fallacy that has existed for years—the sick need to be fed. It is a popular misconception. Researchers are now saying that thousands have been and are being fed into premature graves. It takes bodily energy to digest food, energy that may be needed instead to keep one's heart pumping or one's liver functioning or some other vital organ in operation. Weakness in the sick person is due in most cases not to lack of food, but to a toxic state of the body.[5]

The Mirror of Your Stomach

The tongue is considered to be the mirror of the stomach. The more one's tongue is coated before and during a fast, the more indication that the body needs a total housecleaning. Gradually, as I have related from my own experience, as the body rids itself of these toxins, the tongue will return to a healthy, pink condition. Such a result indicates that you have been on nature's operating table without the use of a knife!

Internal impurity or invisible waste, call it by whatever name you wish, the body accumulates it, and in one form or another, it is eventually going to show itself in an onslaught of disease, physical ailments, discomfort, and yes, aging. The Bible tells us, for good reason, that the blood is the life of man and animals. In recent years we have seen a proliferation of books and other materials written to alert the public to the need to be ecology-minded. Presently, there seems to be a growing interest in the need for public awareness of the need for an ecology with regard to the human body. I, for one, applaud this interest.

The Vehicle of Life

Cleansing and rebuilding the blood stream is ever the first step in working with God to achieve success in any program aimed at reconditioning, healing, and defending our health. Since the human blood stream is the vehicle of life, it must be kept well-nourished and cleansed. Common sense dictates that when the body is healthy, it is less prone to disease. How can one go about ridding the body of that which is disease-producing? The answer is to free up one's elimination systems through the total cleansing brought about by fasting.

Science shows that germs invading the body seek some

type of rubbish heap. When these germs land on toxin-laden cells where the environment is satisfactory for growth, the result will be a sick body in one form or another. Is it any wonder we have physical problems? We have loaded our bodies and digestive tracts with a myriad of laxatives, aspirin, pain killers, prescription drugs, and foreign substances, thereby providing the perfect environment for sickness. Our eating habits are invitations to ill health. In the enlightened age in which we live, and in particular in the kind of life-style that this country boasts of being able to provide for its citizens, you would think we would be the healthiest people in all the world. Unfortunately, this is not true.

Some interesting facts about your blood highlight the necessity to keep this lifeline free of toxic substances that can accumulate:

- We have said before that an individual is as old as his arteries.
- Degeneration and weakening of the arteries shortens life.
- The largest item the body needs is oxygen.
- Oxygen is carried by the red blood corpuscles.
- Each corpuscle is about 1/3200th of an inch in diameter.
- The blood contains from twenty-five to thirty trillion corpuscles.
- Total combined surface of the corpuscles is almost an acre.

In the healthy functioning body, the blood is free of all toxic material. Body wastes pass off through the lungs, the bowel, the skin, and the kidneys.

- During moderate activity, all the blood in the body passes through the lungs more than one hundred times an hour.

- In direct ratio, as the blood becomes stagnant, impure, and abnormal, all organs and parts of the body will decline in health.
- Toxic products in the blood, not time, produce the senile changes called old age.

Do you better understand now the importance of ridding the body of impurities? It is the body that makes the blood and purifies it. It has been wisely pointed out that not even the greatest chemist in all the world can make a drop of blood. Purge the blood of its impurities and the blood can become a flowing fountain that can issue forth in good health, longer life, and a more youthful vitality.

A wise doctor has stated: "The only sickness which exists in the body is toxicity. Healthy cells, nourished properly with organic living food, are immune from such attacks."[6]

The role of proper nutrition in control and prevention of disease has not always been emphasized. In recent years, however, more emphasis has been focused in this area, and new scientific observations are beginning to confirm what many have suspected for some time. Proper eating is extremely important to good health. Fasting can be one of the most effective ways of ridding the body of years of accumulated poisons and aiding in general restoration of health.

6

The Bible Teaches Fasting: Part 1

It should be emphasized that there are those who practice periodic fasting for strictly physical reasons. They make no pretense of fasting for any reason other than that they have discovered its benefits to them from a health standpoint. I have no quarrel with that. But then there are those who know the biblical teachings on fasting and who approach the subject and the practice from that perspective. This is most commendable and certainly to be encouraged. As I have (and will) consistently emphasized throughout this book, a combination of these reasons is most desirable.

Fasting should not be considered a major biblical doctrine nor the answer to every physical ailment. There needs to be a proper balance in our understanding of the subject. It is a subject, however, that the church has neglected for many centuries. It would seem that the secular world has rediscovered the benefits of fasting from a physical and mental sense, whereas many twentieth-century Christians have ignored the biblical teachings. Why this neglect of a teaching that is scattered throughout both the Old and New Testaments, a teaching that always so clearly shows how God moved in response to fasting and praying?

"When our minds are conditioned by prejudice or paralyzed by traditional views, we may face a truth in Scripture again and again without its ever touching us.

Our spiritual inhibition concerning that truth permits us to see, but not to perceive. The truth lies dormant within, mentally apprehended but not spiritually applied. This is particularly true in relation to fasting."[1] I find myself agreeing with writer Arthur Wallis who made this discerning analysis.

What is it that keeps an individual from doing what he knows should be done? The Bible explains:

> For we know that the law is spiritual: but I am carnal, sold under sin. For that which I do I allow not: for what I would, that do I not; but what I hate, that do I. . . . for I know that in me (that is, in my flesh,) dwelleth no good thing: for to will is present with me; but how to perform that which is good I find not. For the good that I would I do not: but the evil which I would not, that I do. Now if I do that I would not, it is no more I that do it, but sin that dwelleth in me. I find then a law, that, when I would do good, evil is present with me. For I delight in the law of God after the inward man: But I see another law in my members, warring against the law of my mind, and bringing me into captivity to the law of sin which is in my members. O wretched man that I am! who shall deliver me from the body of this death? I thank God through Jesus Christ our Lord. So then with the mind I myself serve the law of God; but with the flesh the law of sin (Rom. 7:14,15; 18–25).

Here the apostle Paul eloquently wrote about man's carnal nature. In chapter seven of Romans he showed the inner conflict; in chapter eight he proved that there is deliverance through Christ and consequently no condemnation.

The Spirit Is Life

While Paul is not speaking here specifically about eating habits, the teaching is applicable to *anything* that supplants the working of the Spirit in us.

> For they that are after the flesh do mind the things of the flesh; but they that are after the Spirit the things of the Spirit. For to be carnally minded is death; but to be spiritually minded is life and peace. Because the carnal mind is enmity against God: for it is not subject to the law of God, neither indeed can be. So then they that are in the flesh cannot please God (Rom. 8:5–8).

The teaching is very plain, and as we think about it from the standpoint of physical health, we cannot get away from the implications. We can be slaves to our passions and lusts—including food—or we can sell out to what the Bible teaches and ". . . ye have your fruit unto holiness, and the end everlasting life" (Rom. 6:22). There are definite physical, mental, and spiritual benefits to be derived from obedience to the Word. Fasting is one of those biblical principles that we have neglected. The apostle Paul spoke of fasting elsewhere in unmistakable words.

Immediately upon his encounter with the Lord on the Damascus road, Paul (then called Saul), "was three days without sight, and neither ate nor drank" (Acts 9:9, NASB). Paul knew the teachings about fasting from the Old Testament—knew that this was a practice approved by God and which in time's past brought God's favor—and it is entirely probable that this is why he abstained from eating and drinking. Three days later Paul was seeing *and* "took food" (v. 19).

The record of the early New Testament church in the Book of Acts shows ample evidence that prayer and fasting were very much a part of a deepening relationship with God through the work of the Holy Spirit.

What About the Old Testament Record?

What did Paul and the first Christians know about fasting from the Old Testament record?

Moses, the Lawgiver, the man who saved the nation of Israel from perishing in the wilderness, was known to have achieved mighty results through fasting. Leading the Israelites out of Egypt and bondage was but one of Moses' remarkable achievements; his successors perpetuated his memory by the telling of the giving of the tables of the Law. But first there was that long, lonely vigil on Mount Sinai during which Moses "did neither eat bread nor drink water" (Exod. 34:28). For forty days and forty nights, God and Moses communed. Who among us can imagine what a blessed time that must have been! Yet Moses was human. As such his stomach must have growled, especially the first few days.

When Moses came down from the mountain with the two tables of stone in his hands "written with the finger of God" (Deut. 9:10), he was confronted with a catastrophic crisis—the people once again had rebelled against God and were worshipping a golden calf. Shaking in anger, Moses, threw down the two tablets of the Law, breaking them before the eyes of the people. He feared God's anger and displeasure against the people, knowing that God would be justified in destroying them for yet another inexcusable rebellion.

What did Moses do next? "Thus I fell down before the Lord forty days and forty nights, as I fell down at the first; because the Lord had said he would destroy you. I prayed therefore unto the Lord, and said, O Lord God, destroy not thy people and thine inheritance . . ." (Deut. 9:25,26).

It was back to the mountain for Moses and another time of fasting and praying. There had been no intermission in between; there is no record that Moses had anything to eat or drink. It is believed that this is the longest fast in the Bible, eighty days without food or water. This is considered a supernatural fast. At the end of that time Moses returned. He could say, "I stayed in the mount, according to the first time . . . and the Lord hearkened unto me at that time also, and the Lord would not destroy thee" (Deut. 10:10).

Does prayer and fasting bring results? We have the Old Testament record of Moses to show that they do.

Intermittent days of fasting are related in other Old Testament passages—times of abstention after which it is clearly evident that the hand of God moved in behalf of the fasters.

Women ought to appreciate the reference to the godly Hannah who, with her husband Elkanah, went up to the tabernacle of the Lord and wept and prayed "and did not eat" (1 Sam. 1:7). Her motives were pure. Hannah was childless. Hannah longed to be a mother. So earnest was her prayer that the prophet Eli thought her to be drunk (v. 13). She answered, ". . . No, my lord, I am a woman of a sorrowful spirit: I have drunk neither wine nor strong drink, but have poured out my soul before the Lord. . . . out of the abundance of my complaint and grief have I spoken . . ." (vv. 15,16).

We know that Hannah was the mother of Samuel. But what we so often forget is that God responded to Hannah's prayer and fasting before Him "and the Lord remembered her" (v. 19).

The lesson is plain. We do not come before God fasting just for favors; we come before Him praying and fasting because He is a just and holy God. God will honor our seeking in the way that He knows is best for us. But fasting is a discipline that is pleasing to the Father.

One-Day Fasts Were Common

There were many things that prompted the ancient Israelites to observe one-day fasts. Particularly notable are their days of fasting in repentance for sinning, as in the case of the gathering together at Mizpeh under Samuel's leading (1 Sam. 7:6). They also fasted in times of defeat.

Surely the slaughter of eighteen thousand men in battle would bring any people to their knees in prayer and fasting (Judg. 20:26). A son's grief over ill-treatment of a friend caused Jonathan to rise from the table and refuse to eat (1 Sam. 20:34). Shortly before his death in battle, King Saul observed a one-day fast (1 Sam. 28:20). When David learned of Saul's death, he tore his clothing, as did the men who were with him, "And they mourned, and wept, and fasted . . ." (2 Sam. 1:12).

The murder of Saul's son, Abner, caused David to abstain from eating for a day (2 Sam. 3:35). Uriah, the valiant man of war and husband of Bathsheba, refused food when David called him in from the battlefield (2 Sam. 11:11). David's ruse failed and Uriah ended up a dead hero. Perhaps Uriah was acting more out of sympathy for his comrades than actually fasting, but in view of the Old Testament attitude towards fasting, it would seem that such abstention from food was in keeping with their fasting practices.

God Takes Fasting Seriously

A very somber story is told in 1 Kings 13 where failure to observe a fast that the Lord had declared to a prophet brought tragic death. It is an account of one prophet lying to another prophet thereby causing the second prophet to break his fast. God's judgment fell.

Wicked motives conspired with greed and a scheming woman's plan to obtain property for her husband, and a fast was declared (1 Kings 21:9). The result was the stoning to death of an innocent man, Naboth, and wicked Queen Jezebel's plot to gain a vineyard for her husband, Ahab, materialized.

Elijah the prophet sought out Ahab and unflinchingly pointed out the enormity of his wickedness. Ahab repented, and to show true remorse, fasted and wore sackcloth (v. 27). God deferred judgment because Ahab humbled himself with fasting.

Surely this should say something to the reader as to how God regards fasting *and* repentance!

Fasting Before Battle

Fear of their enemies compelled men like Jehoshaphat and Ezra to proclaim a fast (2 Chron. 20:3; Ezra 8:21). God hearkened to their fasting and praying, and through Jahaziel, the Spirit of the Lord came, and the Lord said, ". . . Be not afraid nor dismayed by reason of this great multitude; for the battle is not yours, but God's" (2 Chron. 20:15).

Those are familiar words—"the battle is not yours, but God's"—uttered frequently by Christians in one way or another to encourage and uplift a downhearted soul. They were originally spoken as God moved in response to prayer and fasting and changed the very course of history.

Fasting Meant Mourning and Humiliation

Mourning for personal sin, mourning for the corporate sins of the congregation (church), and mourning for sins of the nation are all reasons for self-humbling in repentance and contrition. The lessons are there for us in the Bible. We see this in Ezra the priest (Ezra 9:5, 10:6); and in Nehemiah, the king's cupbearer, who was also a former governor, and who became noted for rebuilding the walls of Jerusalem (Neh. 1:4; 9:1).

Fasting Because of Pain and Sickness

In previous chapters I have written about fasting and the beneficial effects this can have upon the body in times of pain and sickness; the Bible shows us in the story of Job's friend, Elihu, how he spoke of abhorring bread and meat while suffering pain (Job 33:20).

The psalmist, David, tells of humbling himself with fasting in times of sickness (Ps. 35:13), affliction, and distress (Ps. 102:4).

Wrong and Right Motives Examined

Usually, when the subject of fasting is discussed by those who are familiar with some of the biblical teachings, there is an immediate reference to Isaiah 58. Here we clearly see that blessings follow obedience to God when such obedience is rightly motivated. Verses 3 to 5 carry a rebuke for wrongly motivated fasting:

> Wherefore have we fasted, say they, and thou seest not? wherefore have we afflicted our soul, and thou takest no knowledge? Behold, in the day of your fast ye find pleasure, and exact all your labors. Behold, ye fast for strife and debate, and to smite with the fist of wickedness: ye shall not fast as ye do this day, to make your voice to be heard on high. Is it such a fast that I have chosen? a day for a man to afflict his soul? is it to bow down his head as a bulrush, and to spread sackcloth and ashes under him? wilt thou call this a fast, and an acceptable day to the Lord?

A selfish fast supposedly for religious reasons prompted by only pride and self-interest was worse than no fast at all. God could not accept it! This fasting was just a form. There was no spiritual outflow from the heart. Although religious zeal was manifested, the proper motive wasn't behind it. Their hearts were not right, and it was actually a mockery to God.

The New Testament carries a similar rebuke for the pharisaical way of fasting (Matt. 6:16; Luke 18:11,12). This is a parading of one's so-called piety merely for the attention and applause of men. Jesus showed His abhorrence for this practice.

Verses 6 through 8 of Isaiah 58 speak of the acceptable fast.

Fasting to Receive Skill and Understanding

If any one biblical figure demonstrated the importance of fasting and praying, it was Daniel. In his beautiful prayer for the people of Israel, the goodness and wholesomeness of the man is seen (Dan. 9). "I set my face unto the Lord God," he said with meekness becoming a man of such integrity, "to seek by prayer and supplications, with fasting . . ." (v. 3).

Quickly, even while he ". . . was speaking, and praying, and confessing *my* sin and the sin of my people Israel, and presenting my supplication before the Lord my God . . ." (v. 20, italics mine), the angel Gabriel came and touched Daniel (v. 21), "he informed me, and talked with me, and said, O Daniel, I am now come forth to give thee skill and understanding. . . . for thou art greatly beloved . . ." (vv. 22,23).

In our "modern" age we seldom hear of angel visitations and ministrations like that! Could this be because we do not demonstrate the sincerity of our commitment through fasting and prayer as Daniel did? Daniel fasted and prayed, and the mighty hand of God *moved.*

Fasting Can Result in Fruitfulness

Another oft-quoted verse of Scripture is found in Joel 2. It is a call to repentance and fasting, but while it is frequently read, the exhortation to fasting is seldom reinforced by pulpit proclamation.

> Therefore also now, saith the Lord, Turn ye even to me with all your heart, and with fasting, and with weeping, and with mourning: And rend your heart, and not your garments, and turn

unto the Lord your God: for he is gracious and merciful, slow to anger, and of great kindness, and repenteth him of the evil (vv. 12,13).

God is saying, in effect, "Show me that you mean business, and I will prove myself gracious, merciful, and all the other things that you so desperately need and desire. Demonstrate that you are seeking me with all your heart," the Lord entreats, "and you can be sure you will be heard on high."

It should be emphasized that prayer with fasting is not going on a hunger strike designed to force God's hand and get our own way, but the idea here presented by the prophet Joel is that of expressing our earnestness in a divinely appointed way. *God's Word says it, I believe it, and I'll do it.* Such fasting—with right motives—will surely result in fruitful living and, even as the book of Joel demonstrates, God's response and the keeping of His promises.

Fasting Can Save a City From Destruction

It was the preaching of a one-time runaway prophet, Jonah, that brought an entire city to its knees in repentance. With his message of woe, the reluctant Jonah, fresh from the belly of the great fish, aroused the king and his nobles to proclaim a fast: ". . . Let neither man nor beast, herd nor flock, taste anything: let them not feed, nor drink water: But let man and beast . . . cry mightily unto God: yea, let them turn every one from his evil way, and from the violence that is in their hands. Who can tell if God will turn and repent, and turn away from his fierce anger, that we perish not?" (Jon. 3:7–9).

We are told "the people of Nineveh believed God, and proclaimed a fast. . . . And God saw their works . . ." (vv. 5,10), and the city was spared.

This spectacular deferring of God's judgment upon a

thoroughly evil city shows God's willingness to move on the behalf of those who take the first step back towards pleasing Him. This extension of His mercy gives great cause for hope to those of us who see nothing but impending doom on a society that presently is so morally bankrupt. That is one of the reasons for the writing of this book. God has put no limitations upon His mercy nor His power. The time for fasting and prayer with repentance is now!

Fasting Was Prescribed by Law

The Old Testament Law prescribed one fast a year, on the Day of Atonement; but later, by the time of the priest and prophet Zechariah, there were at least four a year (Zech. 8:19). Other fasts were frequently called for by the prophets and by the nation's leaders. The problem with prescribed fasting was that it degenerated into virtually meaningless ritual, it became a form of godliness without power, and we shall see Jesus addressing himself to this. Zechariah came along and spoke the Word of the Lord to the people reproving them for such insincere fasting (Zech. 7).

Three- and Seven-Day Fasts

God's ancient people fasted for various periods of time. There are references to three-day fasts as we see Esther instructing her people to do prior to carrying out her bold plan to gain favor from the king and thus spare the life of her people (Esther 4:16).

The death of Saul and his sons caused the valiant men of Jabesh-gilead to steal in by night, take down the bodies of Saul and his sons from the walls, and return them to Jabesh and bury them there. Following that daring feat, they fasted seven days (1 Sam. 31:13).

The story of David and Bathsheba is familiar to most Bible readers. Bathsheba was Uriah's wife; in a moment of passion and weakness, David went to Bathsheba while Uriah was away fighting in battle. "And the woman conceived . . ." (2 Sam. 11:5). Later, Uriah was killed in battle through a wicked scheme of David's. Bathsheba and David were married, and she bore him a son. ". . . But the thing that David had done displeased the Lord" (2 Sam. 11:27).

Later, when this son was struck with a very serious illness, David ". . . besought God for the child; and David fasted . . ." (2 Sam. 12:16). This went on for seven days after which, upon the child's death, David arose and broke the fast (vv. 22,23).

Ten-Day Partial Fasts

When Daniel purposed in his heart that he and his friends would not defile themselves with the king's rich foods and wine, he requested an opportunity to prove his point (Dan. 1:12). For ten days they existed on only beans and water. "And at the end of ten days their countenances appeared fairer and fatter in flesh than all the children which did eat the portion of the king's meat" (v. 15). They were better looking.

Still later, we read of Daniel in mourning for three weeks during which time he ate no bread, ". . . neither came flesh nor wine in my mouth . . . till three whole weeks were fulfilled" (Dan. 10:3).

Another Forty-Day Fast

I shall conclude my references to Old Testament fasting by pointing to Elijah the prophet, surely one of the greatest characters in all the Bible. Elijah boldly challenged the prophets of Baal by calling down fire from heaven, thus turning the tide of apostasy. It was a tremendous answer to prayer as God showed Himself powerful.

It is almost unthinkable that after such a demonstration of almighty power that a man's courage should fail him. But fail him it did, and Elijah starting running for his life. It's incredible, but it happened (1 Kings 19:3). And what is almost worse, Elijah expressed a suicide wish: "... he requested for himself that he might die; and said, It is enough; now, O Lord, take away my life ..." (v. 4).

Elijah needed food. An angel touched him, and there in the middle of nowhere, was a cake baked on coals. There even was a provision of a cruse of water (v. 6). Food fit for angels—provided by the angel of the Lord (v. 7). Elijah went on for forty days in the strength provided by that food and the obvious demonstration of God's power again on his behalf (v. 8). This was a supernatural fast comparable to that which had happened to Moses and later would happen to Jesus.

I believe it is safe to say that fasting revolutionized the life of Elijah. When one studies the Word of God, he learns that the deeply spiritual men who obtained great things in answer to prayer always came through on an empty stomach. These men made history!

Elijah is a case in point. He made history by proving that none of God's children should ever fear potentates, false prophets, and perilous times if their faith is in the true and living God. The lack of food posed no hinderance to Elijah. He endured with a triumphant, conquering faith.

There is no reason why the same cannot be your experience.

7

The Bible Teaches Fasting: Part 2

When you study the biblical references to fasting, you soon notice an emerging pattern, a recurring rationale that explains the underlying motive and, therefore, the reason why the fasters were able to fast with such success.

It's Not What We Do, but Why

Anna, the prophetess, ". . . served God with fasting and prayers . . ." (Luke 2:37).

The leaders of the church at Antioch ". . . ministered to the Lord, and fasted . . ." (Acts 13:2).

The apostolic ministry of Paul was characterized by frequent fastings; He often spoke of the denial of self by forsaking food. In Romans 14:17, for instance, while Paul did not say "don't eat," he did emphasize that there are things more important than eating. "For the kingdom of God is not meat and drink; but righteousness, and peace, and joy in the Holy Ghost."

Jesus talked of fasting (Matt. 6:16–18; 9:14,15; 11:18; 17:21), and He demonstrated prior to entering His public ministry the power that comes to those who are willing to separate themselves from earthly entanglements to seek God's face through prayer and fasting (Matt. 4:1,2 and Luke 4:1,2). This almost six-week period of fasting was preparation for the work that lay ahead, a consecration of Himself to doing the will of the Father.

In all of these references, both in the Old and New Testaments, we see this same consecration on the part of the fasters that marked Jesus' life. It was an absolute turning of one's back on something so insignificant as food as they confronted the far greater need to satisfy the cravings of the inner man in giving of themselves to God in worship and praise.

Because Jesus was both divine and human, we can look upon his fasting days in the wilderness and recognize that the battle waged against Satan was as real as the conflict we will face when we determine to be wholly consecrated to the Father. But we have the assurance both by Christ's example and the promises of the Word that in seeking to worship God, and in serving Him only, God will minister to our needs (Matt. 4:10,11).

We see this too in the example of Paul and Barnabas at the outset of their apostolic ministry:

> As they ministered to the Lord, and fasted, the Holy Ghost said, Separate me Barnabas and Saul for the work whereunto I have called them. And when they had fasted and prayed, and laid their hands on them, they sent them away (Acts 13:2,3).

How different it is today! Often prior to departure of an individual or a couple on a missionary endeavor, a preaching ministry, or entrance into some special aspect of Christian work, friends and family members will get together for a going-away party. Such farewells are more often than not characterized by plenty of food and fellowship. This is not to belittle that practice and the loving efforts put forth by those who mean well, but it is to show how nineteen centuries later we have departed in practice from that which marked the first missionary send-off.

The early church marked the ordination of elders in their work by prayer and fasting (Acts 14:23) and then commended them to the Lord.

One hesitates to ask the question, but in keeping with

the intent of this book the obvious needs stating: What power is much of the local church being denied today, what spiritual vigor would we experience, if as a corporate family led by our leaders, we were to follow the practice of the early New Testament church and address ourselves to days of worshipping the Lord with fasting and prayer?

Stepping from Bondage Into Power

The Bible is filled with references to the great battle being waged between the flesh and the spirit. This is a continual warfare variously described as between the "old man" and the "new man." Paul talked of it as being between good and evil, the natural and the spiritual, between the lower forces and the higher, the earthly and the heavenly, the corruptible and the incorruptible, between the proud and the meek, between intemperance and temperance, and between what is right and what is wrong. The apostle spoke of the necessity of keeping the flesh under subjection:

> Every man that striveth for the mastery is temperate in all things. . . . But I keep under my body, and bring it into subjection: lest that by any means, when I have preached to others, I myself should be a castaway (1 Cor. 9:25,27).

One glance at the average church today gives ample evidence that the body is not being kept under subjection. The Bible talks of our sins of overindulgence in eating as "gluttony," and the moral, ethical, and spiritual precepts that are to characterize the earthly walk of a heavenly-minded people are set forth:

> Be not among winebibbers; among riotous eaters of flesh: for the drunkard and the glutton shall come to poverty . . . (Prov. 23:20,21).

Doctors talk of it in terms of *obesity*. *Gluttony*. *Obesity*.

We shy away from such terminology. Our mishandling of the bounties our Creator has given to us is as much in error as our mishandling of the Word by failing to appropriate its teachings into daily life. We have not recognized that by stepping out of bondage to food we will step into a new freedom and power in the Spirit. There will be a release of energy and an unrestrained joy that will be far more satisfying than our food orgies.

In His beautiful discourse on the mount, Jesus outlined His teaching on fasting and spoke of the need for not being anxious about food and the necessities of life. He directed that there be a "firstness" in our lives:

> Seek ye first the kingdom of God, and his righteousness; and all these things shall be added unto you (Matt. 6:33).

This kind of a perspective would revolutionize our lives. Such a modification of our life-styles calls for a rethinking of priorities. Are we prepared? How do we go about it?

Applying the Principle

Fasting is a method of renewing the mind. I have personally seen it work. I have seen gossipers go on a fast and be cured of a "long tongue." I have seen hot-headed, fiery Irishmen become sweet and gentle. Fasting helps to remove evil thoughts, pride, jealousy, malice, greed, lust, and many other sins of the flesh. Fasting acts as a refining fire. "Let this mind be in you, which was also in Christ Jesus" (Phil. 2:5).

As it pertains to fasting, what was in Christ's mind?

Jesus often taught by comparison. When He discoursed on the subject of fasting, He told His hearers what *not* to do.

> Moreover when ye fast, be not, as the hypocrites, of a sad countenance: for they disfigure their faces, that they may appear unto men to fast. Verily, I say unto you, They have their reward.

But thou, when thou fastest, anoint thine head, and wash thy face; That thou appear not unto men to fast, but unto thy Father which is in secret: and thy Father, which seeth in secret, shall reward thee openly (Matt. 6:16–18).

Notice that Jesus didn't speak of His own experience in fasting; He didn't use Himself as the perfect example of what to do and how to go about it. He cautioned His listeners about an outward display of piety, calling to their attention a disgusting practice of the hypocrites of their day. Pride was their motivation; a totally unacceptable and repulsive motive. So contrary is this to what God desires that Jesus amplified on it in another teaching session when He gave the parable of the Pharisee and the publican:

And he spake this parable unto certain which *trusted in themselves that they were righteous,* and despised others: Two men went up into the temple to pray; the one a Pharisee, and the other a publican. The Pharisee stood and prayed thus with himself, God, I thank thee, that I am not as other men are, extortioners, unjust, adulterers, or even as this publican. I fast twice in the week, I give tithes of all that I possess. And the publican, standing afar off, would not lift up so much as his eyes unto heaven, but smote upon his breast, saying, God be merciful to me a sinner. I tell you, this man went down to his house justified rather than the other: for every one that exalteth himself shall be abased; and he that humbleth himself shall be exalted (Luke 18:9–14, italics mine).

Let's look at that word *humble*. Did Jesus' followers get the message? Did they understand? What did Peter learn? He later said:

. . . be clothed with humility: for God resisteth the proud, and giveth grace to the humble. Humble yourselves therefore under the mighty hand of God, that he may exalt you in due time (1 Pet. 5:5,6).

And what did James gain? His words:

Humble yourselves in the sight of the Lord, and he shall lift you up (James 4:10).

If there is one garment the Christian can do without, it is the *cloak of piety*. We must go back to the hallmark teaching on fasting, Isaiah 58, prophetic in nature, and listen to what the old prophet expounded.

Wherefore have we fasted, say they, and thou seest not? wherefore have we afflicted our soul, and thou takest no knowledge? Behold, in the day of your fast ye find pleasure, and exact all your labors. Behold, ye fast for strife and debate, and to smite with the fist of wickedness: ye shall not fast as ye do this day, to make your voice to be heard on high. Is it such a fast that I have chosen? a day for a man to afflict his soul? is it to bow down his head as a bulrush, and to spread sackcloth and ashes under him? wilt thou call this a fast, and an acceptable day to the Lord (vv. 3–5).

You call that fasting? the prophet is saying. Not on your life! That is nothing short of brazen conceit and God abhors it. The mind set that we must develop, if we are to apply the principle that Jesus taught, is a recognition of our dependence upon a power beyond ourselves to enable us to do for ourselves what mere outward show can never accomplish.

Paul calls this *crucifixion*. We would like to run from that word also, but it is a love-inspired, love-mastered, and love-driven force that will produce the spiritual results we so desperately need. "And they that are Christ's have crucified the flesh with the affections and lusts" (Gal. 5:24).

A lust for food has sent many an individual to an early grave: a grave dug with a fork.

If you will throw yourself upon the mercy of God, seeking His best for your life, then fasting as a means of crucifying your fleshly lust for food, at stated intervals in your experience, can have great physical and spiritual benefits.

The apostle spoke of fasting in regard to one's relationship with a husband or wife. So convinced was he of the benefits of fasting and praying that he enlarges upon this as a help to one's marital situation (1 Cor. 7:5). This is mastery of the physical by the spiritual. Consent of the opposite partner in such abstinence should be obtained. Any effort to satisfy any one of the "carnal appetites" at the time of an extended fast, whether it is the appetite of hunger, sex, or fleshly desire, will mitigate and retard the victory. I do not believe that Paul meant that it would be sinful for a couple to indulge their sexual needs while one or the other was on a fast, but the idea is here presented that greater spiritual results might be felt if, in this also, restraint were exercised for a time.

Purity Among Believers

It is becoming a recognized fact that many illnesses and diseases are caused by eating the wrong foods and by overeating. There is more sickness among overweight people than among those whose weight is normal. Could it be that we have neglected the teaching of 1 Corinthians 10:31 to our own detriment? "Whether therefore ye eat, or drink, or whatsoever ye do, do all to the glory of God."

Can God be glorified in overeating? Can God be glorified by eating or drinking foods and liquids that we know are injurious to our health?

And what do we do with the teaching of 1 Corinthians 6:13?

> Meats for the belly, and the belly for meats: but God shall destroy both it and them. Now the body is not for fornication, but for the Lord; and the Lord for the body.

Elsewhere Paul spoke of the necessity for possessing his vessel in sanctification and honor.

Surely a part of our problem in the Christian church today relates to the emphasis we have placed on the doctrine of grace to an almost exclusion of an equal emphasis on matters relating to discipline. It is as though many theologians and pastors have entered into a conspiracy of silence on this very important subject.

How is the purity of believers to be regained in the affluent society in which most of us live today? Are we sensitive at all to the plight of millions in other places who know nothing of going to bed on a full stomach? Jesus did not totally shun the good things of life while He was here on earth—we read of the times of fellowship He had with friends. He is not asking that we give up such pleasures or that we forego the satisfaction of good food. But how shall we respond to human need in others, and the needs we ourselves have to a more committed life of caring and wanting to be yielded to the will of God in all areas? I believe we need to give earnest consideration to the biblical teachings on fasting.

We need the benefits and blessings that are brought about through fasting and prayer, and the discipline this will require. It surely must grieve our Lord that many of His children have never fasted one day in their entire lifetime. Many would never think of fasting even three days, let alone seven, twenty-one or twenty-eight days. Could this be one of the contributing reasons for a lack of power in our experience? Some scoff at the teachings of fasting in the Bible, declaring them to be outmoded for today. However, when you have done it and have experienced the physical and spiritual blessings that result, your perspective is different.

8

Think on These Things

Have you ever stopped to think that food was involved when man first got into trouble with God? The story is told in the third chapter of Genesis, the opening book of the Bible. It is as sad a story as any recorded in the entire Word of God.

Adam and Eve were morally upright, but they had been given the freedom of choice by their Creator. The garden into which God had placed them was exquisite beyond our imagining. There was no lack of provisions for their every need. Only one prohibition was placed upon Adam and Eve—every tree, shrub, and fruit was theirs to enjoy except ". . . the fruit of the tree which is in the midst of the garden . . ." (v. 3). "The tree of the knowledge of good and evil" was the only exception and would have posed no problem had it not been for the tempter, the devil himself, in the form of a serpent.

Switching to the New Testament, we hear Jesus speak of Satan as being a liar, and the father of lies (John 8:44). Eve did not have the advantage of Jesus' words in Matthew 4:10 where we are told that when Satan tempted Jesus while He was fasting, Jesus said: ". . . Get thee hence, Satan: for it is written, Thou shalt worship the Lord thy God, and him only shalt thou serve."

So Satan, as the seducer in the form of a slithering snake, deceived Eve with a cunning that the devil still uses today. The fruit of the tree took on a new significance to

Eve. She was an unsuspecting victim—innocent, guileless, and certainly no match for her wily antagonist—and she took her first step into self-deception. This is always a dangerous place to be; it is fertile ground for the enemy of our souls. Eve's sisters and brothers have been stumbling into sin ever since. Oftentimes they do not stumble, they rush headlong.

But it was the lure of food and the hoped-for opportunity to "be like God" that brought about original sin. How easily mankind forgets. Food has been the downfall for more than one of God's unsuspecting created beings from that time onward.

Of the Fall in the Garden of Eden, Matthew Henry wrote:

> It was a most dangerous snare to our first parents, as it tended to alienate their affections from God, and so to withdraw them from their allegiance to him. Thus still the devil draws people into his interest by suggesting to them hard thoughts of God, and false hopes of benefit and advantage by sin. Let us therefore, in opposition to him, always think well of God as the best good, and think ill of sin as the worst of evils: thus let us resist the devil, and he will flee from us.[1]

Let us be assured in our own minds that the devil's menu is not in our best interests. If we will venture back to that paradise existence in which our first parents found themselves, we will see that God gave elemental instructions to Adam and Eve as to what should constitute their diet. I am in agreement with those who believe it is in mankind's best interests to look to the ground and what it contains and produces to sustain life. Wade and Hosier, in their book *Eating Your Way to Good Health,* state: "If the all-wise Creator made the first man from the ground, then obviously all the elements in the soil necessary for the building of a body were there to begin with. God in His infinite wisdom neglected nothing."[2]

God has established perfect law and order in the system of nature. Mankind has violated this order and has been suffering the consequences ever since. In the previously mentioned book, the authors take you on a quick trip through the Bible and point out what the Word of God outlines as the way to eat to keep our bodies in maximum health and working order. This, in combination with current knowledge from the field of nutrition, shows the reader how to gain good health from a balanced diet. And fasting has its place. We are reminded of Luke 5:34 and 35. Jesus said to His followers: ". . . Can ye make the children of the bridechamber fast, while the bridegroom is with them? But the days will come, when the bridegroom shall be taken away from them, and then shall they fast in those days." Christ, our Bridegroom, is now taken away. It would appear that His children, in particular, should consider fasting from time to time.

Are you experiencing weight problems? Have you tried every known diet under the sun and experienced nothing but failure? Have you dieted only to gain it all back after a few months? Are there unfulfilled needs in your life or in the lives of family members, friends, your church, or in the lives of business associates? Are you wondering why your prayers aren't being answered? Jesus has provided the clue as to why we are often so ineffective: ". . . this kind goeth not out but by prayer and fasting" (Matt. 17:21). He was specifically referring to casting out of a demon in this instance, but the greater teaching is that there is no substitute for a believing faith that issues forth in prayer and fasting.

The disciples had been unable to cast out a demon from a child. They asked Jesus why they hadn't been able to do this. Jesus told them what the problem was. ". . . Because of your unbelief [little faith]: for verily I say unto you, If ye have faith as a grain of mustard seed, ye shall say unto this mountain, Remove hence to yonder place; and it shall remove; and nothing shall be impossible unto you" (v. 20). There followed the statement about prayer and fasting.

Now that is not difficult to understand. What could be more plain? These are simple words and a simple teaching. Our faith combined with prayer and fasting will open the windows of heaven to bring the power of God into action on the behalf of God's children. And surely this would include ourselves. Such prayer and fasting will bring glory and praise to God when done in the right spirit.

When you pray, fast, and concentrate on "feasting on heavenly manna"—reading the Bible and letting the Holy Spirit indwell your entire being—then stand ready to draw on the limitless resources of your heavenly Father, because it is the Father's pleasure to respond to His children.

Can you imagine being given a check made out to you by a multimillionaire and then *not* cashing it? We are just as foolish in our relationship with God when we are in right-standing with Him through His Son and are not drawing on the resources available to us.

Paul said, ". . . in fastings often . . ." (2 Cor. 11:27). He urged that we keep the old man dead and our lives "hid with Christ in God" (Col. 3:3). We are to crucify the flesh (Gal. 5:24). I have found fasting to be one of the best methods to keep the flesh subdued; it is a restraint that I need to exercise from time to time to bring myself back to the place where I am reminded of these and other verses of Scripture. When we fast in this manner, like the prophet Jeremiah of old, we will discover that God's words are able to sustain us and become as food to our hungry souls. Jeremiah spoke of eating them, and they were the joy and rejoicing of his heart (Jer. 15:16,17). "Oh," you say, "I could never do that. You'd have to be some kind of mystic or have lived in Jeremiah's day to experience that. That's not for us today." I don't find any dates in the Bible that clearly say these references to fasting were only meant for a specified period of history.

Spiritual Benefits of Fasting

The spiritual benefits of fasting can be summed up as follows: (There may be other spiritual benefits you will gain, but these are what I and others have experienced.)

1. Fasting is a discipline of the body in order to humble the soul. David said: "I chastened my soul with fasting . . ." (Psalms 69:10).
2. Fasting helps prevail in prayer with God. "So we fasted and besought our God for this: and he was entreated of us" (Ezra 8:23). When we are willing to set aside the appetites of the body to concentrate on prayer, it demonstrates that we mean business.
3. Fasting with prayer may bring mercy from God, rather than judgment "[The Lord says:] '. . . Turn to me now, while there is time. Give me all your hearts. Come with fasting, weeping, mourning. Let your remorse tear at your hearts and not your garments.' Return to the Lord your God, for he is gracious and merciful . . ." (Joel 2:12,13).
4. Fasting may free us from weaknesses of the flesh such as smoking, drinking, drugs, unnatural sexual desire, and even what Christians consider lesser sins, such as fears, resentment, lying, jealousy, and so on. "Is not this the fast that I have chosen? to loose the bands of wickedness, to undo the heavy burdens, and to let the oppressed go free, and that ye break every yoke?" (Isaiah 58:6).
5. Fasting may free us from bondage to Satan and give us power over him: ". . . In my name shall they cast out devils . . ." (Mark 16:17).
6. Fasting may reveal the will of God for our lives to us. It was when Peter ". . . became very hungry, and would have eaten . . ." (Acts 10:10), that God gave

him the vision that led to the bringing of the Gospel to the Gentiles.

7. Fasting helps us overcome the desire for excessive amounts of food. Paul said:

> I can do anything I want to if Christ has not said so, but some of these things aren't good for me. Even if I am allowed to do them, I'll refuse to if I think they might get such a grip on me that I can't easily stop when I want to. For instance, take the matter of eating. God has given us an appetite for food and stomachs to digest it. But that doesn't mean we should eat more than we need. Don't think of eating as important, because some day God will do away with both stomachs and food.
>
> 1 Corinthians 6:12,13

8. Fasting helps produce the fruit of the spirit—self-control (Galatians 5:22–25; 6:8; Philippians 4:5). When there is failure to deal with the lust for food, one's life is open to attack along other lines. God said of Israel, ". . . when I had fed them to the full, they then committed adultery . . ." (Jeremiah 5:7).

9. Fasting must not be allowed to degenerate into an outward form lacking spiritual value. Christ taught that fasting is a personal matter in the light of needs and circumstances. We are expected to fast, as shown by Christ's statement in Luke 5:34,35.[3]

All These Rewards!

Isaiah 58 is considered by those who practice and recognize the value of fasting as being the classic passage in the Bible on the subject. To read this carefully is to see that the acceptable fast is the one which God chooses (v. 6).

Righteous behavior issues in rewards; but over and over again *we are cautioned that this must not be the motivation.*

I have heard of a woman evangelist who uses a little spoon to say to people, "If this is the way you give to God, then this is what He is obligated to give back to you: 'Give and you will get.' " That is utter nonsense. This same evangelist then proceeds to use a large spoon to illustrate that when we give to God in heaping measure, He is going to repay in same. She then proceeds to elaborate on the need to support the "ministry" of her husband and herself.

Always remember, God looks at your heart; He, and He alone, has the X-ray vision, as it were, that enables Him to weigh motives.

As this relates to the subject of this book, when we choose to fast unto God, according to the directives of His Word, then the promise is that ". . . light shall break forth as the morning, and thine health shall spring forth speedily: and thy righteousness shall go before thee; the glory of the Lord shall be thy rereward" (Isa. 58:8).

This is what can properly be called *acceptable fasting.*

9

Lessons from History

We are creatures of habit. We are also greatly influenced by traditional views. This being true, we are easily prejudiced. We find ourselves approaching subjects about which we have some built-in reservations with preconceived ideas. Our inhibitions prevent us from testing new truths. We may mentally assent to something as being worth investigating, but we fail to venture forth to make application of the truth in our own experience. It's okay for someone else, but it's really not okay for me.

By now you should be convinced that fasting is a practice that merits your consideration. Your conditioning may be such, however, that even though you have been confronted with truth, you haven't allowed yourself to be touched by it. From a physical standpoint, fasting holds promise of yielding real benefits. There is the biblical record that shows fasting to be a mental and spiritual exercise that brought help and hope to those who fasted and prayed to the Lord. It is not too difficult to see that fasting done with the proper motives is pleasing to God.

There is also the record of fasting as practiced by men throughout history. Not only have great saints of church history practiced fasting and testified to its value, but there are lessons to be learned from other historical characters and individuals from the more recent past. Contemporary men and women have documented their experiences with fasting; the records can be examined.

One of the best books on the practice of fasting and its historical background was written by Eric Rogers and is entitled *Fasting, The Phenomenon of Self-Denial.*[1] Rogers reminds us that fasting is as old as prehistory and as new as this week's headlines. Certain practices of fasting have their roots in animism and magic, but every major religion either encourages or requires its followers to practice some form of fasting. It is safe to say, however, that most present-day Christian churches do not emphasize the need for periodic fasts, and many earnest Christians have never even given the subject any serious thought. While it is true that fasting is not considered a major biblical doctrine, nevertheless, when exercised with a pure heart and a right motive, fasting may provide us with a key to unlock doors where other keys have failed. It can be a window opening up new horizons in the unseen world, a spiritual weapon of God's providing.[2]

The Talmud Teaches Fasting

A Jewish fast lasts roughly twenty-six hours, from before sundown until after the next sundown. This is *total* fasting. There are some Jews who observe modified forms of this fast—no food but water. Because the Jews are scattered all over the world, their religious observances of fasts vary. But fasting to the devout Jew is an important part of his compact with God. It signifies a time to express mourning; it provides an expression of repentance and a sign of oneness with all other Jews who share in the covenant.[3]

Early Practices of Self-Denial

Christianity came out of Judaism; therefore, there were many sacred observances, which included fasting practices, that became a traditional part of early Christian church life. Such fasting was done privately (for the individual's benefit) and collectively (to mark events on the church calendar). Historians confirm that fasting was widely approved, rigorously required (by some church authorities), and extensively practiced by the Middle Ages.

As with so many religious practices, the temptation existed for the observance of fast days to deteriorate into mere form or a show of outward piety. This outward pretense and exhibition of holiness was already much in evidence among Jews before Christianity came along. This fasting, followed by feasting, was more for pleasure than for spiritual discipline. This displeased a holy God, and it is to this that Jesus alluded in Matthew 6:16–18, Matthew 9:14–17, Mark 2:18–22, and Luke 5:33–38. Originally, there was much special significance in fasting, but the religionists of Jesus' day greatly overdid it. In every age, we see this happen, not only with regard to fasting, but with other religious observances that start out as being so meaningful and God-blessed. We see then that fasting as a means to advertise one's holiness is forbidden by the Word of God.

In Israel the Day of Atonement (Lev. 16) was a general fast day, and special fast days are mentioned in numerous places elsewhere. We must remember that Mosaic law (under which Christ's followers lived) prescribed these days to "afflict your souls" (Lev. 16:29–31; Num. 29:7). Using that terminology, John Wesley said: "Christians who take heed unto their ways, and desire to walk humbly and closely with God, will find frequent occasion for private seasons of afflicting their souls before their Father which is in secret."[4]

In the first centuries of the Christian church, Wednesdays and Fridays were fast days.[5] Pharisaism had introduced two fasts weekly, on Mondays and Thursdays, and has has already been pointed out, it was the pharisaical practices that Jesus condemned. It can be seen, however, that from the beginning two days were set apart as fast days, a practice that showed the dependence on Judaism, although clearly a protest is evidenced by the change of days.

As you trace the history of fasting, particularly down through the early church, it is amazing to see the temper of the times displayed. Anti-Jewish feelings flared with the Jews celebrating Saturdays as festival days, and Christians dishonoring them by fasting!

Fasting for Christians was to be based in principle upon the sufferings of Christ. In the time of the apostle Paul, no definite Christian custom seems to have existed.

> One man esteemeth one day above another: another esteemeth every day alike. Let every man be fully persuaded in his own mind. He that regardeth the day, regardeth it unto the Lord; and he that regardeth not the day, to the Lord he doth not regard it. He that eateth, eateth to the Lord, for he giveth God thanks; and he that eateth not, to the Lord he eateth not, and giveth God thanks (Rom. 14:5,6).

Paul, it can be seen, is setting before the Roman Christians the ideal mind set. One can readily sense the controversy that must have been waging among those early Christians as to what days they were to observe. As one reads those words, you get the feeling that Paul was close to being irritated about these frustrating matters. (Read the verses that follow; they are very significant.) Paul wanted the Christians to get on with holy living, demonstrating a Christ-like spirit, and he strained to get that important point across.

> For the kingdom of God is not meat and drink; but righteousness, and peace, and joy in the Holy Ghost. For he that in these things serveth Christ is acceptable to God, and approved of men. Let us therefore follow after the things which make for peace, and things wherewith one may edify another (vv. 17–19).

As you study the history of fasting in the early church, you see to what extremes they went as they tried to justify why they fasted on certain days. Legendary explanations would have one believe that the apostle Peter greatly influenced the thinking of the church at Rome with regard to religious observances—including fast days. But the Roman customs did not spread widely.

Resistance to fasting grew among early Christians. More than likely, this came about because of the hypocritical attitude of those who practiced it for self-righteous reasons. Fasting was always meant to be a channel of power, but as true spirituality waned and worldliness flourished in the churches, those who understood Jesus' teachings and the apostle Paul's warnings withdrew from any outward show of fasting. This is not to say these old-time saints were not practicing it in private; we have reason to believe that they were, and that some of God's saints through the ages have always fasted. (See Chapter 6.) An examination of the journals and biographies of some of the church's great saints shows that these individuals persevered in prayer and fasting before the Lord, and the church moved forward as God honored their deep contrition and temporary devotion of all their energies to prayer and spiritual communion.

Hippocrates Fasted

It usually comes as a something of a surprise for people to discover that Hippocrates, often called the "father of medicine," fasted. It was he who wrote: "Abstinence and quiet cure many diseases."

Hippocrates was the outstanding physician of his time. He was born about 460 B.C. Hippocrates had a wise teacher, Herodicus, who taught his student that diet and exercise were of far greater value to one's body and health than drugs or medicines. Consider, will you, that this was in the fifth century B.C.!

Hippocrates's success was so notable that rulers from as far away as northern Greece and Persia came to him for help. The textbooks and records he left for posterity were unequalled for over seventeen hundred years. And what did the physician recommend primarily? Hippocrates believed that *nature* was the best healer. The Hippocratic Oath on ethical medical practices is still used by medical graduates today.

Other Famous Fasters

Tertullian wrote in A.D. 210 that fasting was a better aid to religion than feasting.

Polycarp said in A.D.110 that fasting was a powerful aid against temptation and fleshly lusts.

Socrates and Plato fasted periodically. Fasting among the Greeks was quite common, as it was among the Egyptians and the Druids. Arameans, Arabs, and Ethiopians fasted. Fasting is found in most primitive religions from the Esquimaux of Alaska to the Aborigines and Maoris of Australasia.[6] It is not surprising that fasting was (and still is) very common in oriental religions. One thinks immediately of Ghandi of India.

History shows that many have been made "saints" for the asceticism of their diet.[7] One cannot help but wonder, however, if the extremes of food deprivation to which some of these went actually convinced others of the spiritual benefits, or whether these acts of mortification only succeeded in putting a kind of superstitious fear in observers.

The rigidity of the demanding asceticism in the early centuries of the Christian era saw many monks and hermits subjecting their bodies with a misguided and intemperate zeal to ruthless forms of repression. All excessive fasting that would injure the body or in some manner interfere with the true practice of Christianity as outlined in the *whole* of the New Testament is to be avoided. Fasting that requires spectators or approval by others is not true fasting. Jesus instituted *no* fasts for His first disciples.

The disciples had both the record of the Old Testament men and women and generations of tradition handed to them; therefore it was not necessary for Jesus to institute new dates for fasting nor explain to them the way it was to be done. What He did say, however, is very significant. After telling them what *not* to do, He added, "But thou, when thou fastest, anoint thine head, and wash thy face" (Matt. 6:17). Notice that He didn't say, "*If* you fast." Clearly, the Lord took it for granted that His followers *would,* and one can add, I believe, *should* fast. What Jesus was emphasizing was that they should go on about their business and affairs as usual. Our religious practices are never to be for the sake of impressing others but rather an expression of our heart to the Father.

Fasting in the early church fell into many abuses. The danger of this happening always exists. The fact that Jesus did not set up a new system for fasting may have had something to do with His foreknowledge of future events. He knew a new day for Christianity was about to dawn. The old system, even as the book of Hebrews so beautifully explains, was just a shadow of the good things that were yet to come (Heb. 10).

Much of the fasting practiced under the old Jewish system was tied to a rigid legalism. Jesus explained it so well when He said that we should not sew new cloth to an old garment, neither do you put new wine into old bottles (Matt. 9:16,17). As it pertains to fasting, the implication was that there would be a new dimension to their reasons for fasting. We are living in the age of the church, that is the period of the absent Bridegroom. "And Jesus said unto them, Can the children of the bridechamber mourn, as long as the bridegroom is with them? but the days will come, when the bridegroom shall be taken from them, and then shall they fast" (Matt. 9:15).

The disciples' and our reasons for fasting periodically today should be, among other things, an actual act of preparation as we look for Jesus' return. Linking all of the Old Testament and New Testament teachings on the subject, it should not be difficult to understand that now is the time for periodic fasting as we wait for that blessed reappearing of our Lord.

Fasting in the medieval Christian church was done primarily on Fridays to commemorate the death of Jesus. Following the principle of fasting before feasting, the church observed fasting before Christmas, Epiphany, Pentecost, and Easter. Customs varied from church to church and from country to country. For those who practiced it properly, there was undoubtedly great spiritual blessing. One custom, which was early emphasized in connection with fasting, is worthy of special attention—the giving of alms and provisions to the poor, from the money saved because of fast days, brought help and hope to the needy. Surely this practice is in keeping with helping the world's hungry today, and one that the Christian church could well afford to copy.

Some strange fasting ordinances came into existence. In the sixth century, for instance, fasting was no longer voluntary. The Council of Orleans, 541, declared all who failed to keep the stated times of abstinence to be offenders against the laws of the church. Then in the seventh century, the Council of Toledo issued a summons that those who ate meat during Lent were unworthy to partake of the resurrection.

By the time the eighth century rolled around, fasting was considered meritorious and offenders against fasting ordinances were excommunicated. And, can you imagine, in some cases people had their teeth knocked out for eating meat during Lent!

Lenten fasts became common (forty days before Easter). It was largely a modified form of fasting, however, with the emphasis mainly being on one meal a day, and this was to be as simple as possible. The idea was to limit the enjoyment of food to the barest necessities, or to refrain from certain designated articles of food. It was not actually until the 1960s, when the Catholic church underwent major changes in liturgy and other religious observances, that rules regarding Lenten fasts were relaxed. This brought to an end nearly two thousand years of dietary restrictions.[8]

Fasting and the Reformation

It is not surprising that the great Reformers practiced fasting and testified to its value as a spiritual exercise. The journals of these men reveal that they took seriously the biblical injunctions to fast and pray.

The practice of fasting crossed denominational lines; theology, it would appear, was neither a deterrent nor did it make fasting obligatory. We see Luther, who had so recently come out of Catholic dogma with its many rituals to which he objected, finding peace in his monastery at Erfurt. While praying and fasting he had read the Word and meditated upon it. One day the meaning of God's forgiveness through Christ came to him like the sun bursting through clouds after a rain, and Luther was never the same again. After that experience, Luther periodically fasted while translating the Bible. It was he who cautioned against the church's stringent demands for self-denial that led people to think they could justify sin and immorality by fasting. He rightly emphasized that it was not Christ's intention to reject or despise fasting but to restore proper fasting.

Many of the early Reformers fasted- and prayed-down

what has since been called the "Old Time Power." They did not make a great "to-do" about it, and so it was not widely known that God was moving, among other things, in answer to the faithfulness of these men of God who were literally following what Jesus said in Matthew 17:20 and 21. (See Chapter 8.) Fasting is, in a sense, like faith, and the number of those who understand both are not as great as one might suppose.

Jonathan Edwards, the great American theologian and preacher of the 1700s, practiced fasting. John Calvin, whose views were generally adopted by the Reformed churches, commended the practice of fasting but cautioned against doing it for superstitious reasons.

The Westminster Confession says that "solemn fastings" are "in their times and seasons" to be used in a holy and religious manner.[9]

John Wesley, energetic founder of the Methodists, was a fervent faster. Throughout his lifetime he preached in favor of fasting. In times of national or spiritual crisis, public leaders and pastors have called for fast days. There is record of Wesley calling for such a fast on Friday, February 6, 1756. The open Bible was Wesley's guide, and he was only following in the stead of the likes of King Jehoshaphat (2 Chron. 20:1–4), Ezra (Ezra 8:21–23), and calling to remembrance what happened to Nineveh as a result of Jonah's preaching (Jon. 3).

Wesley wisely cautioned against excesses in fasting; yet in so doing, he called for its practice. Wesley knew from first-hand experience, there was an acceptable course to follow. In the somewhat stilted and formal English of his day, Wesley's famous sermon on fasting speaks to the same problem that rears its head for us in this age. But we need to hear what this man of God had to say:

> First, let it be done unto the Lord, with our eye singly fixed on

Him. Let our intention herein be this, and this alone, to glorify our Father which is in heaven; to express our sorrow and shame for our manifold transgressions of His holy law; to wait for an increase of purifying grace, drawing our affections to things above; to add seriousness and earnestness to our prayers; to avert the wrath of God; and to obtain all the great and precious promises which He hath made to us in Jesus Christ. . . . Let us beware of fancying we *merit* anything of God by our fasting. We cannot be too often warned of this; inasmuch as a desire to 'establish our own righteousness', to procure salvation of debt and not of grace, is so deeply rooted in all our hearts. Fasting is only a way which God hath ordained, wherein we wait for His unmerited mercy; and wherein, without any desert of ours, He hath promised freely to give us His blessing.[10]

John Knox fasted; Rees Howells was a faster. Robert Chapman of Barnstaple spent every Saturday fasting. Someone who called on him on that day said,"His face shone as the face of an angel."

David Brainerd and Charles Finney knew what it meant to observe the gentle art of fasting. We learn also that Pastor Hsi of China and Pastor Blumhardt of Germany—both men whom God used mightily in the deliverance of those bound by Satan—were regular fasters. These men are representative of some of the great scholars and preachers of times past who knew the value of fasting.

Andrew Murray, whose meditative writings have enriched the thinking of multiplied thousands, wrote:

Fasting helps to express, to deepen, and to confirm the resolution that we are ready to sacrifice anything, to sacrifice ourselves to attain what we seek for the kingdom of God.[11]

One of the great Bible commentators of all time, Matthew Henry, wrote:

Fasting is a laudable practice, and we have reason to lament it, that it is so generally neglected among Christians.[12]

A writer of our generation, D. Martyn Lloyd-Jones, has stated:

I wonder whether we have ever fasted? I wonder whether it has even occurred to us that we ought to be considering the question of fasting? The fact is, is it not, that this whole subject seems to have dropped right out of our lives, and right out of our whole Christian thinking.[13]

Early Settlers in America

Because of the heritage of their European ancestors, many of America's early settlers spent solemn days in fasting. Ministers of the first colonies actively promoted the observance of fast days. These days were observed with scrupulous religiousness after the manner of the Puritan Sabbaths.[14]

This is not to say that many of these early settlers were not in earnest about these fast days with hearts that were right before God. The hand of God moving on their belief can be seen in the pages of history. Surely prayer and fasting played a part in such divine intervention.

Reformer-fasters

I have already called attention to the fasts of Ghandi, entertainer Dick Gregory, and novelist Upton Sinclair. This country, in recent years, has seen its share of what someone has called "reformer-fasters" who have walked across the stage of life and through publicized fasts have dramatized the plight of one group or another. We can point, for instance, to Cesar Chavez, Mexican-American labor leader. Such hunger strikes are not uncommon in the United States as well as elsewhere.

Scientists and Health Advocates

In efforts to attain dietary reform, men and women

scientists and health advocates have gone on fasts. It is not denied that many current food fads are detrimental to one's health. In the process of trying to inform one's self, the need for caution must be emphasized. Many books and articles call for fasting, but you are well advised to proceed with care. For further enlightenment, specifically read *Fasting, The Phenomenon of Self-Denial,* by Eric N. Rogers (Thomas Nelson, 1976), pages 107–124.

Another book that is worthy of close examination is entitled *Fasting Can Save Your Life*, by Dr. Herbert M. Shelton. Splendid results through supervised fasting have been obtained under his direction. I have frequently referred to Dr. Paavo Airola's books. These men, dedicated to hygienic living, are considered fasting experts. While these and other writers do not always agree as to method, they are in agreement as to the value, particularly from a health standpoint, of periodic fasting.

10

"How Do I Begin a Fasting Program?" and Other Frequently Asked Questions

The key to success in almost any endeavor is mental discipline. Impatience has rung the death knell on many a venture. As this relates to one's decision to embark upon a fasting program, or an altered eating pattern to improve one's health, the need exists to in effect "psych" one's self out so that you are thinking not in terms of food deprivation, but of an ultimate goal that is going to be far more rewarding and satisfying than any immediate gratification food could provide.

This is *not* an unbiblical concept. At one place in the Bible, as the apostle Paul addressed the Corinthian Christians about giving to other Christians, he spoke of the necessity for first having "a willing mind." In another place, this same apostle urged the development of the kind of mind set that Jesus had: "Let this mind be in you, which was also in Christ Jesus" (Phil. 2:5). Still later, Paul asked the Philippian believers to ". . . think on these things" (Phil. 4:8), and he gave them an array of things on which to focus that would help them realize their greatest God-given potential. The point is that the Bible shows us the importance of the right kind of thinking whenever we embark upon ventures that are going to be different from the norm.

Good-bye to Fear of Failure

Fear of failure is a major reason why so many people

never succeed at a new venture. They just simply give up before they even give themselves a fair start.

The conscious mind, we are told, can hold only one thought at a time. If we consciously program ourselves to think success, we will succeed. How can you do this? Visualize yourself the way you wish to be:

healthy
energetic
bright-eyed
at your ideal weight
pleasant to be around
exercising faith
spiritually receptive
mentally alert

These and other attributes are associated with vim, vigor, and vitality. Health and normal weight, (taking into account your height and skeletal structure) do go hand in hand.

Dr. Bernard Jensen, world traveler, lecturer, nutritionist, longevity philosopher, author, and researcher, has spent his lifetime studying natural methods for attaining and retaining health and vitality. In his book, *World Keys to Health and Long Life,* he shows how those who develop the greatest amount of activity—physically, mentally, and spiritually—and who get the most, therefore, out of living, are those who treat their bodies well. For the most part, these are people who are healthy and joyous as they live in tune with nature. The people who live the longest are those who practice disease prevention, Jensen has discovered. The philosophy of too many people today is to take for granted the measure of health they possess, and then when they get sick or have other problems, they go to the doctor and hope he can help.

Dr. Jensen's travels have taken him to parts of the world where men and women live to be 120 and even older. Some of these people still have beautiful teeth when they die, and their bodies are remarkably preserved. Fasting is a way of life for such people and is done at stated intervals (often in conjunction with religious practices), such as one day a week. For many there is total abstention (defined as water only) during the fast; others use juices.

The old men and women whom Dr. Jensen visited had one quality in common—they were wise and sparing in their actions. They were prudent in carefully administering to their bodies just what they knew those bodies could handle. This meant they didn't extend their bodies beyond what they knew they could repair or rebuild.

Economy in the Body

Overeating and overindulgence consume vital bodily energies. In time this will wear out the body. Doesn't it stand to reason then that giving these bodies an opportunity to periodically rest is a form of body energy conservation? When there is a great reduction in the amount of food consumed, our digestive, glandular, circulatory, respiratory, and nervous systems have a chance to rest. When no food is taken in, they can rest most of all.

Back to the title of this chapter: *How Do I Begin a Fasting Program?* You begin by being convinced that fasting is a discipline you should cultivate. While you are fasting, it is a good time to educate yourself as to the next step in taking care of your body—the role of proper nutrition. A recommended reading list on nutrition is provided in the back of this book.

No More Munching, Crunching, and Nibbling

If the truth were known, we would be shocked at how many people have formed habits of munching, crunching, and nibbling their way through life. With your decision, however, to embark on a fasting program to cleanse your body, and your new resolve to adhere to this program, comes the necessity to forget food for whatever period of time you have chosen for your first fast. Hold out to yourself the expectation that you can expect an almost immediate weight loss of two, three, or more pounds after the first twenty-four hours. Daily there will be a weight loss and an accompanying feeling of well-being. Hold out to yourself also the expectation that you may very well rid your body of many aches and pains, as some of us can attest happens.

How To Do It

Set a time and begin your fast. You may determine at the outset that your fast will be for a day, three days, or longer. Particularly on the longer fasts, your body will signal when you are exceeding what is best for you. Do not give in to initial hunger pangs, however, and think your body is trying to tell you something—it's objecting, to be sure, but not in the way you think.

It is advisable to prepare yourself for fasting through a two- or three-day cleansing diet. This is best achieved by eating nothing but raw fruits and vegetables—fruits in the morning, no noonday meal, and then a fresh vegetable salad in the evening.

There are some who recommend (at the outset only) a mild laxative to cleanse one's bowel. Others suggest a double enema: First use a pint of plain water, then let it out; second, repeat with a full quart of water into which camomile tea or a few drops of lemon juice have been added.

If you are going on an all water fast, you will need to drink a minimum of two quarts (sixty-four ounces) of water each day. Mineral water, soft spring water, filtered water, or any water free of impurities is acceptable. If you are going on a combination water and juice fast, you can periodically drink juice and then water. The point is that the liquids will help to rid the body of toxic wastes, and the body requires liquids.

There is some difference of opinion as to the need to take enemas throughout the fast. Dr. Airola, considered to be one of the world's leading exponents of fasting and an authority on how to get well and stay well, believes enemas during fasting are a must. Dr. Shelton, on the other hand, believes enemas to be irritating (see *Fasting Can Save Your Life,* page 68). I have found personally that an enema every four or more days did no harm. This is something you will have to determine for yourself.

To help you better understand some of the conditions that may arise, particularly during an extended fast, one needs to be forewarned. By recognizing these conditions and understanding their meaning, concern and alarm can be alleviated. There are some difficulties that may arise, especially during an extended fast of more than a few days' duration.

Simply Put, What Is Fasting?

Fasting is simply abstinence from food; it is not abstinence from all of the other essentials of life. And this is abstinence only in the sense that we abstain from food for a period of time. Fasting is allowing the body to draw on its stored-up supplies. Fasting is not suspended animation; we do not go into hibernation like some animals do. It is important that our bodily functions continue and that all our other bodily needs are met.

Some Things You May Experience

In a previous chapter I told you of my own symptoms during a fast; you will undoubtedly experience early hunger pangs, a growing acidosis accompanied by a bad taste in the mouth, some body odors, headaches, and a lightheaded or dizzy feeling at times. In addition, you may have some bowel problems—I have found that enemas do relieve these.

On several of my fasts, I have been bothered by hiccups. This is caused by a spasmodic contraction of the diaphragm. It is usually caused by bile in the stomach or sometimes by intestinal obstruction. I have found the sucking of an ice cube brings relief. The tightening of a belt around the waist, gradually increasing the pressure, will also assist in remedying the condition.

At the beginning and near the end of the fast, you may feel more weakness. This is to be expected, it is a lassitude that is not unnatural to fasters. This weakness will be more pronounced if drugs have been used in large quantities in the past, and also by those who smoke and consume large amounts of coffee. It is always felt by the alcoholic, and is usually felt by those who for long periods have been overeating. One of the best ways to overcome this problem is to take walks, breathe deeply of the fresh air, and avoid strenuous exercise.

What About Exercise?

Your body needs as much oxygen as possible in order to aid in the cleansing process that is taking place in your system. This is necessary to hasten the regeneration and revitalization process. Walking and mild exercise are recommended, but an overexpenditure of one's strength is not advised.

There were times while I was fasting that I had the feeling of cold feet. If this happens to you, in the privacy of your home or office, walk around on your toes. This aids in circulation and burns considerably more energy than regular walking. If you are sitting still and can't do anything else, wiggle your toes. Even that speeds up circulation and burns up energy.

It is important to keep active during your fast. There are those who mistakenly think one should slow down and rest as much as possible, or more than usual, while fasting. It is important to live your normal life and do your regular work. If you are in a position of employment where you are expending great amounts of energy in physical exertion, you should attempt to take it easier. Someone in this situation would be well-advised to fast under the supervision of a doctor if the fast is to be for any more than a short duration.

On my last fast of twenty-eight days, one time I suddenly got out of bed, and before I knew what was happening, I blacked out and fell backwards onto the bed. Had I not known what was occurring, upon coming to, I would have been greatly alarmed. Such dizziness is not uncommon. What it says to the faster is, do not suddenly stand up. Learn to pace yourself in your movements.

What About Bathing?

The need for cleanliness does not change while one is fasting! In fact, I have found that sometimes it is necessary to take two or three baths a day to be relieved of the strange odors. Jesus said, "But thou, when thou fastest, anoint thine head, and wash thy face" (Matt. 6:17). There is no reason to fear the bad breath and skin odors, but rather rejoice, knowing that the stagnant poisons are being released from your body. Bathing should, however, be of short duration. There are mixed opinions as to the temperature of the water one should use. The body consumes considerable energy in resisting extremes of heat or cold. Bathing during fasting is for cleansing purposes, not for any supposed therapeutic effects. Sponge bathing may be necessary if there is weakness or if the faster is more advanced in age. Some fasters may need help in bathing. Sauna baths during fasting are not something I would recommend.

What About Sunbathing?

As with anything, moderation is to be preferred. But sunshine serves important purposes for plant and animal life, and there are beneficial effects for us humans when we do not overexpose ourselves to the rays of the sun.

Other Things That May Occur.

Sometimes a faster will experience a humming in the head. This is caused by a temporary anemia of the brain, and if this does occur, it will not remain. You may also find an excess of wax excreting from your ears. This may also be the cause of the ringing noises in your head. The excretion of wax is another method the body uses during a fast to eliminate waste.

It is possible that during an extended fast you will feel cramps. These cause pain in the stomach, hands, legs, and feet. I have experienced these on twenty-one- to forty-day fasts. Such cramping is a result of spasmodic contractions of the muscles working in oversensitive nerves. It can be caused by the breaking loose of long-retained fecal material in the colon or the accumulation of gas from such long-held decomposing bowel content.

Sometimes, early in the fast, vomiting may take place or there may be slight nausea without vomiting. This happens more often to an extremely overweight person. This is only an effort on the part of the stomach to eject the filth, poisons, and other accumulations that perhaps have been there for weeks or even months. The nausea or vomiting could also be caused by an unloading of bile from the liver and gall bladder that is frequently caused by reverse peristalsis, which is a flowing backward of bile into the stomach rather than down through the intestinal canal through which it should properly pass. Enemas have been found helpful at times like this. Great relief can be had by drinking warm water, and deep breathing of fresh air. When experiencing acute vomiting, many fasters become frightened and break the fast. If effort is made to break the fast and food still is ejected, once again it would be better not to eat until natural hunger returns and the body retains food without this problem. This occurrence is relatively rare.

Another condition which may occur, although it is infrequent, is some problem with kidney function. More often, people who are troubled with kidney problems will find the condition quickly clearing when fasting is instituted. Dramatic changes have been documented in cases of Bright's disease or nephritis when patients fasted. The body can do incredibly amazing things for itself in the way of restoration and function when given the opportunity.

If you have any problems with urination, drink all the hot water possible. Again, I have found that enemas will help. A very hot bath with the abdomen submerged usually helps the situation as well. Never hesitate, of course, to consult your doctor if health problems seem aggravated by fasting, or if no relief occurs when something does seem to flare up.

Pain in the heart or palpitation is prevalent at times when gas in the stomach presses against the heart. Drinking two or three glasses of warm water soon removes this and gives relief. Sitting or lying down for a few minutes also will help. If this disturbance is only minor and does not continue, there is generally no cause for alarm.

What About Taking Vitamins?

Questions may arise in the minds of individuals who wish to fast about the use of vitamins. Many health-conscious people are sold on the need for supplementing their diets with vitamins. Recognition exists that many of our foods come to us depleted. Millions of us have been jolted out of our complacency by such books as *Eating May Be Hazardous To Your Health*, by Jacqueline Verrett and Jean Carper (Simon and Schuster, 1974), a soberly gripping book that tells of the silent violence in many of our foodstuffs. The need for vitaminizing and mineralizing our bodies exists. So what does a person do about this when he fasts?

Most of the material written with regard to fasting recommends that the intake of vitamins and food supplements should be discontinued completely while on a fast.

What About Drugs?

Drugs also should not be used while fasting. Exceptions would be for those who are taking medication for heart disease, insulin for diabetes, and cortisone for arthritis. But these individuals should not be fasting anyway unless their fast is supervised by an experienced practitioner.

What About Drinking Coffee?

Can you drink coffee while on a fast? The answer is *no.* Smoking and drinking of alcoholic beverages are also forbidden.

Can Everyone Fast?

Fasting is not for everyone. Nursing mothers, diabetics who are taking insulin, and people with terminal illness should not fast. Children should not fast unless medically supervised. If you are troubled with gout, blood diseases, heart disease (especially thrombosis), tumors, cancer, bleeding ulcers, liver and kidney diseases, I believe you should refrain from extended fasts. Such individuals would, I believe, benefit from twenty-four hour or three-day fasts, but beyond that they should seek medical supervision.

An underweight person should never fast more than thirty-six hours, and this only every three months. Again, such an individual is advised to seek medical supervision.

Others who should not go on extended fasts are those with tuberculosis, pernicious anemia, and spinal cord syphilis.

There is some controversy over whether pregnant

women should fast. Dr. Herbert M. Shelton (*Fasting Can Save Your Life*) believes that nausea and vomiting during pregnancy are signals that the woman is toxemic to some degree. The mother's body is going to work to give the unborn child the very best that can be given. Since the unborn child feeds upon substances supplied by the mother, any systemic unpreparedness will cause the mother's body to work to correct the problem. Nausea and vomiting may be part of a general renovating program. This rebellion in the stomach causing it to reject food is the body's command to stop eating. Shelton says it is even more than that: It is a process of purification, a means of freeing the body of accumulated toxins. He is convinced that the pregnant mother who experiences nausea and vomiting will not be harmed by ceasing to eat until she feels better, and neither will the unborn child. When eating is resumed, he cautions that it should be in moderation with a light feeding of fruits and uncooked vegetables. This is one doctor's opinion. The pregnant woman should always consult with her own doctor.

Fasting With Someone Else

A fun way to try fasting is with your wife or husband, or with a co-worker or friend. Each morning when you weigh, compare and rejoice together as you scale down. It can bring real joy as you see your dress size slip from a sixteen down to a twelve and even to a ten. Men can have the same experience by notching in their belts, seeing their stomachs shrink, and feeling their pants get baggy. How nice to have to buy trousers several sizes smaller! How encouraging to stand in front of a full-length mirror and hardly recognize yourself!

Understanding the Cleansing Process

Bear in mind that your entire system is going through a

thorough housecleaning while you are fasting. As long as there is waste material in your circulatory system, you will feel some discomfort during the fast. As soon as this passes through your kidneys you will feel much better. This should explain why you feel better and stronger as you progress in the fast; the more your system becomes unclogged, the more it becomes purified, and the better you should feel.

Professor Arnold Ehret, originator of what he called the "Mucusless Diet Healing System" and long a disciple of health, recommended that his fasters drink water with a little lemon and honey to loosen the mucus in the circulation.[1]

How Long Should You Fast?

Caution needs to be exerted in determining the duration of a fast. Professor Ehret (mentioned above) argues that a fast lasting too long may become detrimental if the sick organism is too greatly clogged up by waste. Fasters have been known to suffocate in their own waste—something that sounds unbelievably ugly. This is particularly possible if an individual has been on prolonged drug usage. To have all this waste material suddenly dumped into one's blood stream may impose too much stress on one's circulatory system. People in this condition may need shorter fasts combined with some eating days of cleansing on what Professor Ehret called a mucusless diet in combination with laxatives and enemas.[2]

A fast under twelve days is considered a relatively short fast. A fast of fourteen to twenty-one days is a medium-length fast; and a fast of forty days is a long fast. One's natural appetite subsides as he continues on a medium or long fast. Daniel, the Old Testament faster, fasted for twenty-one days. He was determined not to be defeated. He kept right on praying and fasting until victory came. It appears from a study of biblical fasters that right motives play an important part in one's ability to sustain a fast of extended duration.

If you are fasting mainly to lose weight, then the more weight you want to lose, the longer your fast must be. You may need, however, to interrupt fasting with eating days of cleansing (described above).

Since we do not accumulate excess weight in a matter of a few days, it stands to reason we will have to work harder to rid ourselves of the fat hanging from our limbs or our middles. In a ten-day fast, one can begin to see some outstanding victories.

The duration of one's fast should be determined by you and you alone. (However, it is recommended that you work with a doctor if you undertake a long fast.) No one is going to force you to go on a total fast. If it is your desire to lose weight, to look better, to feel better, to gain back your self-respect—or if you choose to fast for mental and spiritual reasons—these are choices only you can make as you consider your general health and other factors.

The heart and the stomach work harder than any other parts of our body. Hogs and humans are the only creatures that keep their stomachs loaded twenty-four hours a day. Sometimes an individual lives a whole lifetime without giving his stomach a decent rest.

Go on a hunger strike for the glory of God! Give your stomach a vacation. Some people make their stomachs a big storehouse like the one the Bible's Joseph erected in Egypt. To look at them you'd think they thought it would be seven years before they'd eat again! We are empty of grace and full of grease! Hundreds of churches do not have one member, including the pastor and deacons, who have *ever* fasted. We have become a people who worship athletics and appetites and have forsaken the Almighty.

There are literally millions of people in America who are overweight. Think of it: In a world with millions who are undernourished and dying of starvation, we are stuffing ourselves to death by overeating or by eating the wrong foods. There are many reasons why we should fast—health reasons and physical benefits are surely important motivations. The Christian who fasts usually combines spiritual motivation with recognition that he will be benefited physically as well. But whether one is a Christian or a non-Christian, fasting can also be a commitment to care for a hungry, hurting world. Enough committed individuals like this, would, in time, make a difference. For motivation in this direction, I recommend reading Dr. W. Stanley Mooneyham's book, *What Do You Say To a Hungry World?* Among other practical considerations, Mooneyham recommends that money saved by not eating could be channeled to relief agencies to help people who fast all the time—involuntarily.

There is no excuse why fasting for you should not be a tremendous success. It cannot fail if you obey the rules. In America, we are "food intoxicated." Everytime the television is turned on we see portrayed a choice cut of meat, some "yummy" cake, pie or other goody, a carton of "delicious" ice cream, or an enticing drink. We are a people who have acquired a lust for food. The "hunger lust" has slain many saints. Fasting, I am convinced, could empty many doctor's waiting rooms and thousands of hospital beds.

11

Breaking the Fast

In 1 Samuel 30, there is the story of an Egyptian who had been lying in a field three days. He was found by David's men. His explanation revealed that because he had fallen sick while in battle, his master had just left him (v. 13). When he was brought to David, he was given bread, ". . . and he did eat; and they made him drink water; And they gave him a piece of a cake of figs, and two clusters of raisins: and when he had eaten, his spirit came again to him: for he had eaten no bread, nor drunk any water, three days and three nights" (vv. 11,12).

This fast of the Egyptian had been imposed and certainly not self-chosen. The fact that he was sick to begin with, and then was without water for three days, made him very weak. We see here the care David and his men exercised in helping him regain his strength. They knew what and how to eat after going without food.

Moderation

What this says to us is *moderation*. Caution is needed, especially if the fast has been longer than three days. What you are attempting to do is to bring the body back to normal efficiency with the reintroduction of food. The normal body is going to signal its hunger when the body has used up its store of accumulated reserves. If you think it was difficult to discipline yourself to get through the first few days of an extended fast, then you will also discover that the first few days of coming off a fast require similar discipline.

You have not been in hibernation during the fast, but your bodily organs have been, in effect, sleeping. Gently and slowly you will want to call them back into activity.

It is possible to have some problems if the fast is broken improperly. During the fast the body rids itself of excess water and any bloating will disappear. But if you attempt to break the fast too rapidly or eat the wrong kinds of food, you may encounter bloating again. It is important therefore to begin eating slowly and in the right manner. You cannot be too careful in this regard.

If you encounter any problem with eating after the fast, *stop eating.* If there's difficulty, drink as little water as possible and take an enema. A hot bath is beneficial, and rest and relaxation at this time are in order. Give yourself time to start ingesting solids.

The men whom I have quoted in this book have their own ways of breaking a fast. You may wish to read their materials also and decide what you feel would work best for you. Some fasting experts advise putting a little bulk back into the system to act as sort of a broom to clear out any remaining residue. Dr. Shelton suggests breaking an orange into small sections and eating portions of it every two hours the first day. Professor Ehret suggests eating fresh, sweet fruits, such as cherries and grapes. He also recommends soaked or stewed prunes and even small helpings of raw or stewed vegetables. Dr. Airola has a four-day plan for breaking a fast. He suggests the use of a half apple the first day; soaked prunes or figs the next; the third day a glass of yogurt, a small fresh green salad, and a slice of whole grain bread. However, everyone is in agreement about *moderation.* DO NOT OVEREAT!

What Worked For Me on My Forty-day Fast

I generally end all my long fasting on Welch's grape juice (unsweetened), orange juice (fresh squeezed), or apricot juice. This is my schedule for the days following an extended fast:

Day One

Mix one quart of juice with one quart of mineral water. Drink about a tablespoon of this mixture every few minutes, making sure the half-gallon of mixture lasts throughout the first twenty-four hours after the fast ends.

Day Two

Use one quart of *undiluted* grape, orange, or apricot juice and sip on this for a twenty-four hour period. Divide it into three-ounce portions and slowly sip at two-hour intervals. Drink a minimum of fifty ounces of mineral water also.

Day Three

Take forty ounces of grape, orange, or apricot juice and divide it into ten equal parts of four ounces each. Slowly sip these portions every one and a half hours. Drink a minimum of fifty ounces of mineral water.

Day Four

During the day drink forty ounces of grape, orange, or apricot juice every one and a half hours in four-ounce portions. Mix one grated apple in two cups of plain yogurt. Divide into six equal parts and have one portion every two hours. Drink the fifty ounces of mineral water.

Day Five

Drink the forty ounces of juice in ten four-ounce portions over a two-hour span. Drink the fifty ounces of mineral water. Mix one grated apple, one grated carrot and two cups of plain yogurt. Divide into six equal portions. Have a portion every two hours.

Day Six

Drink one quart of grape, orange, or apricot juice. If you have been drinking grape juice, alternate to one of the others. Take four ounces at two-hour intervals. Drink at least thirty-two ounces of mineral water. Mix one grated apple, one grated carrot, two teaspoons of honey, one teaspoon of lemon juice, and two cups of plain yogurt. Divide into six equal parts and have a portion every two hours. Eat two slices of melba toast anytime you desire, but no more than two slices! Do not break with these allowances at this point.

Day Seven

Drink forty ounces of apricot, grape, or orange juice in five-ounce portions every one and a half hours. Drink a minimum of thirty-two ounces of mineral water. Mix one grated apple, one grated carrot, two teaspoons of honey, one teaspoon of lemon juice, and two cups of plain yogurt. Divide the mixture into five equal parts and have a portion every two hours. Three slices of melba toast can be consumed. This is the day you can add six almonds, walnuts or pecans.

Days Eight to Thirteen

Drink one quart of apricot, grape, or orange juice in four-ounce portions every two hours. Continue drinking at least thirty-two ounces of mineral water, more if possible. Mix the same yogurt mixture and eat over a span of four hours. Eat four slices of melba toast, six nuts (choice of walnuts, pecans, almonds) or ten peanuts. One cup of cooked cereal with milk. One slice of pumpernickel bread. (Add no salt to the cereal.)

Day Fourteen

Drink one quart of orange, grape, or apricot juice in four-ounce servings over two hours. Drink at least a quart of water. Make the same yogurt mix and consume in equal parts over four hours. Six slices of melba toast, six of your choice of nuts or ten peanuts. One cup of cooked cereal with milk. One slice of pumpernickel or whole wheat bread. Six ounces of cottage cheese topped with a tablespoon of sour cream.

Days Fifteen to Twenty-One

Same as previous day. Add to the diet at one of the meals three potatoes pureed in milk with one teaspoon of butter. No salt.

Days Twenty-Two and Thereafter

Use the foods you have been consuming up until this day in moderation, but slowly add other fruits, juices, soups and broths, potatoes, raw or steamed vegetables. If your legs or hands evidence any swelling, cut back on your eating. At that point you may want to go without food for a day or so until this clears up. You will learn to gauge your body's needs.

A build-up of natural and health-promoting foods should gradually be added to your diet. Only then will the healing and regenerative forces begin functioning properly again. You have fasted to clean out your system and to give your vital organs a much-needed rest; do not ruin the effects of all this by lapsing into your old habits.

After the fast pay closer attention to the food on your plate. Among other things, you can reduce the risk of hypertension that often leads to coronary heart disease, strokes, congestive heart failure, and kidney diseases. Salt is a contributing factor in many of these diseases. The average body consumes *ten times* the salt it needs. A thirty-five-year-old woman with blood pressure fifteen percent above normal can add eight or nine years to her life span by sharply reducing salt intake.

We all need to moderate our eating of meat, dairy products, and fried foods. Shift from beef and pork to poultry and fish. The evidence is overwhelming that meat is contributing to much ill health. Use vegetable fats instead of animal fats. Eat more vegetables, fruits, whole grains, and whole grain products. It is important to get enough roughage in our diets to aid in elimination processes.

Drink lowfat milk rather than whole milk. Eliminate as much as possible the use of white sugar and products made with white sugar and white flour.

Unless one is performing heavy manual labor, two meals a day—when properly selected, prepared, and consumed in the right combinations—give ample nourishment. There are some individuals who are finding that one meal a day is adequate. The older a person becomes, the less food one's body requires.

Farmers fertilize their crops with the exact combinations they need. Cattle are given what they require. But humans eat anything and everything, frequently without even thinking about what this is doing to their bodies. We eat and drink, stuffing ourselves with "junk foods" knowing, in the back of our minds, that this is detrimental to our well-being.

In Proverbs 30 we find a prayer request and a confession spoken in the same sentence. Amazing! If only we would remember this every time we stuff something into our mouths: ". . . feed me with food convenient for me: Lest I be full, and deny thee . . ." (vv. 8,9).

It is possible to do this, to feed one's body with foods that are needful and nourishing; but to refrain from eating that which in time will weaken, irritate, and make it sick requires discipline. Additives and seasonings have deadened our tastebuds. You will notice after coming off your fast that those tastebuds are extremely sensitive. This is good and it is in your best health interests that you keep them that way. Reckless eating habits, however, will undo all the good that is derived from a fast.

Limit your caloric intake and resist the temptation to put back into your "refinery" those foods that are only going to impair the proper running of your system.

Our Life Span

You don't need to be told that your possible life span, at best, is really very short. If we lived eight times our growth period, as is the case of many animals, we would have an average life span of 192 years. We drink the same water, breathe the same air, and live under the same sunshine and elements as do the animals. What makes the difference in terms of longevity?

Could it be what we take into our bodies in the way of food and nourishment? We eat too much and too often. That is an established fact. You have now seen what happens to your digestive system and other organs when the burden of too much and improper food is placed upon it. Indigestion, which is usually the first signal that not all is right, is caused by improper chemical reactions of the foods you have consumed. Fermentation and irritation result. We pay for our indiscretions with suffering, pain, and discomfort. Some eventually pay with their lives. And we also suffer spiritual loss—we do not function at our best physically, mentally, or spiritually when our bodies are out of tune.

The Basic Four Food Groups

To receive adequate nutrition on a regular basis, you should remember that a well-balanced diet will include essential nutrients from four basic food groups: (1) milk and its products; (2) meats, eggs, and other protein sources; (3) fruits and vegetables; (4) cereals and their products.

The milk group includes cheese, yogurt, ice cream, and other milk-based foods. Adults are advised to consume two or more glasses of milk daily; children three or more glasses; teenagers and pregnant and nursing mothers four or more glasses. We can get this in ways other than drinking (custard, creamed soups, etc.).

The meat group includes the usual animal foods, but fish, poultry, and eggs are considered part of the meat group. Two or more servings of protein-rich food from the meat group should be eaten daily.

Vegetables and fruits provide abundant sources of roughage needed for good elimination. The importance of fruits and vegetables in the diet of early man can be seen from the biblical record. We would all be better off health-wise if we ate more of our vegetables and fruits raw. You are assured of getting important vitamins and minerals in your diet when you eat "nature's way."

In the *bread and cereal group* one should opt for natural whole-grain varieties that do not contain chemical additives and sugar. When baking, substitute whole-grain flours for white, so-called "enriched" flours. Four or more servings are recommended.

Other Foods

Sugar and sweeteners are not included in the Basic Four; neither are salt and other condiments nor beverages (except for milk and juices). Certain amounts of these, of course, will be consumed. But the reader should think twice before overloading one's system with these things. Remember, sugar has no protein, vitamins, or minerals. The average individual in this country uses from 104 to 170 pounds per year. This is incredible! (Read Dr. John Yudkin's *Sweet and Dangerous* [Bantam, 1973].)

Try using herbs instead of salt and other condiments in your cooking. They are becoming increasingly popular and most gourmet cooks know of their value; now it is up to the average homemaker to recognize their worth.

And what can I say to warn and convince you of the need

to watch your beverage intake? We have become a caffeine-addicted people. Look at these figures:

Coffee—100 to 150 milligrams of caffeine per cup
Tea—about 90 milligrams per cup
Cola drinks (12-ounce bottle)—40 to 72 milligrams
Cocoa—about 50 milligrams per cup

Cancer of the bladder and heart attacks are only two of the problems that may arise for heavy consumers of caffeine beverages.

A growing number of people are victims of a comparatively new health problem—hypoglycemia, or low blood sugar. Carbonated drinks, it has been discovered, are a prime contributing factor. Symptoms include nervousness, irritability, lethargy, insomnia, headache, heart palpitation, irregular heartbeat, some nausea, diarrhea, and other equally disturbing problems.

Accountability to Our Creator

The apostle Paul tells us in unmistakable terms that we are accountable to our Creator:

> What? know ye not that your body is the temple of the Holy Ghost which is in you, which ye have of God, and ye are not your own? For ye are bought with a price: therefore glorify God in your body, and in your spirit, which are God's (1 Cor. 6:19,20).

There is the motivation that should prompt every one of us to break our bad eating habits and consider our accountability to God.

12

The Choice Is Ours

For years people have been in pursuit of what is called the "fountain of youth." It is an elusive thing for most. Dr. Bernard Jensen's research shows that the people who attained longevity had bodies that were not much heavier than they had when they were twenty years of age.[1]

The "fountain of youth" is, for most of us, within arm's reach—right in our kitchens where we prepare our foods, or if we frequent restaurants, we have the choice of taking the menu in hand and making wise choices. We have the option of whether we want a healthier, longer, and more satisfying life, or whether we will settle for second best or worse. But among those choices should be regular periods of abstention from food through fasting. Whether we are doing it for purely health reasons, or mental and spiritual benefits, or a combination of all three, there is sufficient evidence to prove that we can attain our goals.

Fasting connotes pain but also possibility—the possibility of the realization of one's aspirations. The question is: Are you willing to risk the one for the other? The pain is not so much physical as it is the initial mental anguish of turning one's thoughts off of food. Food *is* a celebration; the pain is in giving up this pleasure for a set time.

Choose Life

An often overlooked passage of Scripture that holds

great promise is to be found in the Old Testament book of Deuteronomy. "See, I have set before thee this day life and good, and death and evil; . . . I call heaven and earth to record this day against you, that I have set before you life and death, blessing and cursing: therefore choose life . . ." (Deut. 30:15,19).

The word *choose* is an annoyance to many. Decision-making does not come easy to everyone. But the thing we dislike about the word is what separates us from the rest of God's creation. To choose or not to choose is a gift. We are compelled by God to make choices. From the outset of creation it's been that way, and God has reserved that special gift for us humans.

There is power in this matter of choosing; unfortunately, from the creation account and ever since, mankind has been making unwise choices. And we end up suffering the consequences. God plainly told us to "choose life." The witness of the Old Testament is of a wandering, staggering, miserable people who died to what life could be.

What Real Life Is

Death in the biblical sense is more than physical death. We die daily when we refuse to make choices that can lead to a sense of health and well-being in the here and now. Real living comes when we realize our personal responsibility to determine the direction of our lives. The invitation to "choose life" is an ever present thing. Past failure does not disqualify us; the mistakes of the past do not mean that we are failures as human beings. God calls us continually to new life; He holds out the option of new beginnings. The potential is always there; and so is God's faithfulness to help us realize our goals. There is also the witness in the Old Testament of people who grasped the meaning of listening to God's call for choosing life and its immense possibilities. We know of Moses, Isaiah,

Jeremiah, Abraham, and others. And there is the witness in the New Testament.

But "What If . . . ?"

The common characteristic of those who fail in an endeavor is a "What if . . . ?" attitude.

"What if I make this decision to fast and I can't stick to it?"

"What if I don't have the strength to continue?"

"What if my willpower gives out?"

Many people don't even make it to the "What if?" stage. At least give yourself the benefit of the doubt and make a determined effort to begin.

New beginnings are usually not easy, simple, or comfortable. When you sense that you are about to stumble and give up, call to remembrance God's words: "I set before you life and death . . . *choose life*."

If you are fasting and temptation comes, take an extra long drink of water or juice, look up and claim God's promise to help in your times of need, and turn your back on the temptation to quit.

Respond Positively to God's Invitation

Recognize too that you have an adversary. The Bible calls him by name. The devil is a master of deceit. Satan is full of wiles and evil intent. Do as Jesus did. ". . . Get thee hence, Satan . . ." (Matt. 4:10). Respond positively to God's invitation to life, and know that in the choosing, you have access to His power to prevail.

Practical Considerations

Generally, we all should drink more water. Do you know how much water is contained in living things? Water makes up 95 percent of a jellyfish; 79 percent of a lobster; 65 percent of a kangaroo rat; and 48 percent of a pea weevil. Water comprises 65 percent of the human body.

The human kidney is 82.7 percent water. Water comprises 74.5 percent of the brain, 75.6 percent of muscle, 83 percent of blood, and 22 percent of bone.

A ripe tomato is 95 percent water, a ripe pineapple 87 percent, and an apple 80 percent.

I give you these statistics to nudge you into a realization that water is *very* essential to all plant and animal life. In fasting I have discovered that the more water I drink, the more successful a particular fast will be.

Water helps assuage any momentary feelings of hunger or weakness. Water relieves the "fuzzy" feeling that develops in my mouth. (The fuzziness, remember, is a good sign indicating that toxic poisons are being eliminated. Be thankful for that "fuzzy" feeling.)

Foods to Eat to Keep Your Weight Down

After you have finished fasting, eat these foods in moderation. From this list you can see that you will not be deprived. Retrain your thinking and work to modify future behavior so that you do not lapse into the old habits that created your weight or health problems. Note the weight schedule (at the conclusion of this chapter) and see how you measure up. Fasting is going to help you reach your desired weight.

High Protein Foods

Cottage cheese and hard cheese (American, Swiss, Jack, etc.), yogurt, diet margarine or vegetable oils, eggs, chicken or turkey, beef, veal, lamb, venison, rabbit, fish, oysters, clams, crabs, shrimp, seeds, and nuts.

Low Calorie Vegetables

Asparagus, bean sprouts, green beans, cabbage, cauliflower, celery, cucumbers, green peppers, lettuce, watercress, endive, mushrooms, parsley, spinach and other greens, summer squash, and zucchini.

High Calorie Vegetables

Beets, brussel sprouts, carrots, turnips, parsnips, okra, onions, peas, lima beans, soybeans, tomatoes, winter squash, and pumpkin.

Beverages

Water (of course), low-fat or skim milk, herb teas or decaffeinated coffee (no sugar; if you must sweeten, learn to use honey), bouillon and clear soups, buttermilk, tomato juice, fresh fruit juices (whenever possible) or frozen (preferable to canned).

Fruits

(some of these are higher in calories than others)

Apricots, bananas, berries, cherries, oranges or grapefruit, grapes, pineapple, peaches, cantaloupe, honeydew or watermelon, pears, rhubarb. (Whenever possible eat fruits fresh; if you must eat canned fruits, use those water-packed.)

Breads and Cereals

Whole wheat, rye, pumpernickel, buckwheat pancakes or waffles, granola cereals or other whole-grain cereals not coated with sweeteners.

IDEAL WEIGHT SCHEDULE

WOMEN

Height		Bone Structure		
Ft.	In.	Small	Medium	Large
4	9	92-100	97-110	107-123
4	10	95-103	100-112	110-125
4	11	100-106	103-115	111-125
5	0	101-108	106-117	114-130
5	1	104-110	109-120	117-132
5	2	106-115	112-125	120-136
5	3	110-120	116-128	124-143
5	4	112-121	120-134	130-145
5	5	116-125	124-140	130-148
5	6	120-130	126-142	135-152
5	7	125-135	131-146	140-157
5	8	128-138	135-150	144-162
5	9	132-142	139-156	147-166
5	10	137-149	143-160	152-162
5	11	142-160	148-170	157-170
6	0	145-165	150-175	160-175

IDEAL WEIGHT SCHEDULE

MEN

Height		**Bone Structure**		
Ft.	In.	Small	Medium	Large
5	1	110-120	117-128	125-140
5	2	113-121	120-132	127-144
5	3	117-126	122-137	131-149
5	4	120-130	126-140	133-151
5	5	122-131	130-142	136-157
5	6	126-135	133-146	140-160
5	7	130-140	136-150	148-165
5	8	135-145	141-155	150-168
5	9	137-149	145-160	154-172
5	10	142-152	148-163	157-180
5	11	145-157	152-168	161-185
6	0	150-160	157-174	167-190
6	1	155-167	160-180	170-195
6	2	160-172	166-186	175-200
6	3	163-176	171-190	180-205

Recommended Reading List

Abrahamson, E. M., and Pezet, A. W. *Body, Mind & Sugar.* New York: Pyramid, 1951.

Airola, Paavo, *How To Get Well* and *How To Keep Slim, Healthy and Young With Juice Fasting.* Phoenix: Health Plus Publishers, 1974.

Albright, Nancy, ed. *The Rodale Cookbook.* Emmaus, Pa.: Rodale Press Inc., 1973.

Anderson, Lynn. *Rainbow Farm Cookbook.* New York: Harper and Row Publishers, Inc., 1973.

Bailey, Herbert. *Vitamin E: Your Key to a Healthy Heart.* New York: Arc Books, 1968.

Blaine, Tom R. *Goodbye Allergies.* Secaucus, N.J.: Citadel Press, 1968.

Blevin, Margo, and Ginder, Geri. *The Low Blood Sugar Cookbook.* New York: Doubleday and Company, Inc., 1973.

Braaten, Carl E., and Braaten, LaVonne. *The Living Temple: A Practical Theology of the Body and the Foods of the Earth.* New York: Harper and Row Publishers, Inc., 1976.

Brown, Edith, and Brown, Sam. *Cooking Creatively with Natural Foods.* New York: Ballatine Books, Inc., 1973.

Chen, Philip S. *Soybeans for Health and a Longer Life.* New Canaan, Conn.: Keats Publishing, 1974.

Cheraskin, Emanuel, et al. *Psycho-Dietetics: Food As the Key to Emotional Health.* New York: Stein and Day, 1974.

Cheraskin, E., et al. *Diet and Disease.* Emmaus, Pa.: Rodale Press, Inc., 1968.

Clark, Linda. *Know Your Nutrition.* New Canaan, Conn.: Keats Publishing, Inc., 1973.

Clark, Linda. *Help Yourself to Health.* New York: Pyramid Publications, 1974.

Cleave, T. L. *Saccharine Disease: The Master Disease of Our Time.* New Canaan, Conn.: Keats Publishing, Inc., 1975.

Recommended Reading List

Cott, Allan. *Fasting: The Ultimate Diet.* New York: Bantam Books, 1975.

Cross, Jennifer. *The Supermarket Trap: The Consumer and the Food Industry.* Bloomington, Ind.: Indiana University Press, 1970.

Dankenbring, William E. *Your Keys to Radiant Health.* New Canaan, Conn.: Keats Publishing, Inc., 1974.

Davis, Adelle. *Let's Cook It Right,* rev. ed. New York: Harcourt Brace Jovanovich, 1962.

Davis, Adelle. *Let's Eat Right and Keep Fit.* New York: Harcourt Brace Jovanovich, 1970.

Davis, Adelle. *Let's Get Well.* New York: Harcourt Brace Jovanovich, 1965.

Davis, Adelle. *Let's Have Healthy Children,* new and exp. ed. New York: Harcourt Brace Jovanovich, 1972.

Davis, Francyne. *Low Blood Sugar Cookbook.* New York: Bantam Books, Inc., 1974.

DiCyan, Erwin. *The Vitamins in Your Life.* New York: Simon and Schuster, 1974.

Duffy, William. *Sugar Blues.* Radnor, Pa.: Chilton Book Co., 1975.

Ehret, Prof. Arnold. *Mucusless Diet Healing System* and *Rational Fasting.* Beaumont, Calif.: Ehret Literature Pub. Co., 1975.

Elwood, Catharyn. *Feel Like a Million.* New York: Pocket Books, Inc., 1976.

Ewald, Ellen B. *Recipes for a Small Planet.* New York: Ballantine Books, Inc., 1975.

Ford, Margie, et al. *The Deaf Smith Country Cookbook: Natural Foods from Family Kitchens.* New York: Macmillan Publishing Co., Inc., 1973.

Fredericks, Carlton. *Eating Right for You.* New York: Grosset and Dunlap, Inc., 1972.

Fredericks, Carlton, and Bailey, Herbert. *Food Facts and Fallacies.* New York: Arc Books, 1968.

Fredericks, Carlton, and Goodman, Herman. *Low Blood Sugar and You.* New York: Grosset and Dunlap, Inc., 1969.

Goodwin, Mary T., and Pollen, Gerry. *Creative Food Experiences for Children.* Washington, D.C.: Center for Science in the Public Interest, 1974.

Hall, Ross H. *Food for Nought: The Decline in Nutrition,* new ed. New York: Harper and Row (Medical Department), 1974.

Hightower, Jim. *Eat Your Heart Out: How Food Profiteers Victimize the Consumer.* New York: Crown Publishers, Inc., 1975.

Hunter, Beatrice T. *Beatrice Trum Hunter's Whole-Grain Baking Sampler.* New Canaan, Conn.: Keats Publishing, Inc., 1972.
Hunter, Beatrice T. *Consumer Beware!* New York: Simon and Schuster, Inc., 1972.
Hunter, Beatrice T. *Fact-Book on Food Additives and Your Health.* New Canaan, Conn.: Keats Publishing, Inc., 1972.
Hunter, Beatrice T. *Fact-Book on Yogurt, Kefir and Other Milk Cultures.* New Canaan, Conn.: Keats Publishing, Inc., 1973.
Hunter, Beatrice T., ed. *Food and Your Health.* New Canaan, Conn.: Keats Publishing, Inc., 1974.
Hunter, Beatrice T. *Natural Foods Cookbook.* New York: Simon and Schuster, Inc., 1969.
Hylton, William H. *The Rodale Herb Book: How to Use, Grow and Buy Nature's Miracle Plants.* Emmaus, Pa.: Rodale Press, Inc., 1974.
Jacobson, Michael F. *Don't Bring Home the Bacon.* Washington, D.C.: Center for Science in the Public Interest.
Jacobson, Michael F. *Your Guide to Better Eating.* Washington, D.C.: Center for Science in the Public Interest.
Jarvis, D. C. *Folk Medicine.* Greenwich, Conn.: Fawcett World Library, 1958.
Jensen, Bernard. *World Keys to Health and Long Life.* Escondido, Calif.: Omni Publishers, 1975.
Josephson, Elmer A. *God's Key to Health and Happiness.* Old Tappan, N.J.: Fleming H. Revell Co., 1976.
Kenda, Margaret E., and Williams, Phyliss S. *The Natural Baby Food Cookbook.* New York: Avon Books, 1973.
Kirban, Salem. *How To Keep Healthy & Happy by Fasting.* Irvine, Calif.: Harvest House Publishers, 1976.
Kugler, Hans J. *Slowing Down the Aging Process.* New York: Pyramid Publications, 1973.
Lager, Mildred, and Jones, Dorothea Van Gundy. *The Soybean Cookbook.* New York: Arc Books, 1968.
Lappe, Francis M. *Diet for a Small Planet.* San Francisco, Calif.: Ballantine Books, Inc., 1975.
Larson, Gena. *Fact-Book on Better Food for Better Babies and Their Families.* New Canaan, Conn.: Keats Publishing, Inc., 1972.
Lindsay, Gordon. *Prayer and Fasting.* Dallas, Tex.: Christ For the Nations, Inc.
Mae, Eydie, and Loeffler, Chris. *How I Conquered Cancer Naturally.* Irvine, Calif.: Harvest House Publishers, 1976.
Marine, Gene, and Van Allan, Judith. *Food Pollution: The*

Violation of Our Inner Ecology. New York: Holt, Rinehart and Winston, Inc., 1972.

Martin, Clement G. *Low Blood Sugar: The Hidden Menace of Hypoglycemia*. New York: Arc Books, 1974.

Mooneyham, W. Stanley. *What Do You Say to a Hungry World?* Waco, Texas: Word Books, 1975.

Newman, Marcea. *The Sweet Life: Marcea Newman's Natural Food Dessert Cookbook*. New York: Houghton Mifflin Co., 1974.

Nusz, Frieda. *The Natural Foods Blender Cookbook*. New Canaan, Conn.: Keats Publishing, Inc., 1972.

Ogden, Samuel. *Step by Step to Organic Vegetable Growing*. Emmaus, Pa.: Rodale Press, Inc., 1971.

Page, Melvin E., and Abrams, H. Leon. *Your Body Is Your Best Doctor*. New Canaan, Conn.: Keats Publishing, Inc., 1972.

Passwater, Richard. *Supernutrition: Megavitamin Revolution*. New York: Dial Press, 1975.

Paterson, Grusha D., Editor. *Health's-a-Poppin'*. New York: Pyramid Books, 1973.

Pauling, Linus. *Vitamin C and the Common Cold*. San Francisco, Calif.: W. H. Freeman Co., 1970.

Pfeiffer, Carl C. *Mental and Elemental Nutrients: A Physicians' Guide to Nutrition and Health Care*. New Canaan, Conn.: Keats Publishing Inc., 1976.

Pinckney, Edward R., and Pinckney, Cathey. *The Cholesterol Controversy*. Los Angeles: Sherbourne Press, 1973.

Pomeroy, L. R., ed. *New Dynamics of Preventive Medicine*. 2 vols. New York: Stratton Intercontinental Medical Books Corp., 1974.

Ratcliff, J. D. *Your Body and How It Works*. Pleasantville, N.Y.: Reader's Digest Press/Delacorte Press, 1975.

Robbins, William. *The American Food Scandal*. New York: William Morrow and Co., Inc., 1974.

ɔgers, Eric N. *Fasting, The Phenomenon of Self-Denial*. Nashville: Thomas Nelson, 1976.

Rohrer, Virginia and Norman. *How To Eat Right and Feel Great*. Wheaton, Ill.: Tyndale House Publishers, 1977.

Ross, Shirley. *Fasting, The Super Diet*. New York : Ballantine Books, 1977.

Rosenberg, Harold, and Feldzaman, A. N. *The Doctor's Book of Vitamin Therapy*. New York: G. P. Putnam's Sons, 1974.

Schroeder, Henry A. *The Trace Elements and Man*. Old Greenwich, Conn.: The Devin-Adair Co., 1973.

Selye, Hans. *The Stress of Life.* New York: McGraw-Hill, 1956.
Shelton, Herbert M. *Fasting Can Save Your Life.* Chicago: Natural Hygiene Press, 1975.
Shute, Wilfred E., and Taub, Harald. *Vitamin E for Ailing and Healthy Hearts.* New York: Pyramid Publications, Inc., 1972.
Smith, David R. *Fasting, A Neglected Discipline.* Fort Washington, Pa.: Christian Literature Crusade, 1969.
Spira, Ruth R. *Naturally Chinese: Healthful Cooking from China.* Emmaus, Pa.: Rodale Press, Inc., 1974.
Stone, Irwin. *The Healing Factor: Vitamin C Against Disease.* New York: Grosset & Dunlap, 1972.
Taub, Harald J. *Keeping Healthy in a Polluted World.* New York: Harper and Row, 1974.
Tobe, John H. *The Natural Foods No-Cookbook.* Don Mills, Ontario: Greywood Publishing Limited, 1973.
Turner, James S. *Chemical Feast: Report on the Food and Drug Administration.* (Ralph Nader Study Group Reports) New York: Grossman Publishers, Inc., 1970.
Verrett, Jacqueline, and Carper, Jean. *Eating May Be Hazardous to Your Health.* New York: Simon and Schuster, Inc., 1974.
Wade, Carlson. *Fact-Book on Fats, Oils and Cholesterol.* New Canaan, Conn.: Keats Publishing, Inc., 1973.
Wade, Jean G. and Hosier, Helen Kooiman. *Eating Your Way To Good Health.* Old Tappan, N.J.: Fleming H. Revell, 1977.
Wallis, Arthur. *God's Chosen Fast.* Fort Washington, Pa.: Christian Literature Crusade, 1970.
Watson, George. *Nutrition and Your Mind: The Psychochemical Response.* New York: Harper and Row, 1972.
Wigmore, Ann. *Be Your Own Doctor.* New York: Hemisphere Press, n.d.
Williams, Roger J. *Alcoholism: The Nutritional Approach.* Austin, Tex.: University of Texas Press, 1959.
Williams, Roger J. *Nutrition Against Disease.* New York: Bantam Books, Inc., 1973.
Williams, Roger J. *Nutrition in a Nutshell.* New York: Doubleday, 1962.
Williams, Roger J. *The Wonderful World Within You: Your Inner Nutritional Environment.* New York: Bantam Books, Inc., 1976.
Yudkin, John. *Sweet and Dangerous.* New York: Bantam Books, Inc., 1973.

Notes

Chapter 1

[1]Paavo Airola, *How To Get Well* (Phoenix: Health Plus, Publishers, 1974), p. 214.

Chapter 2

[1]Airola, *How To Get Well,* p. 216.

[2]Ibid., p. 219.

[3]Karen Wise, *God Knows I Won't Be Fat Again* (Nashville: Thomas Nelson, 1978).

[4]Shirley Ross, *Fasting, The Super Diet* (New York: Ballantine Books, 1976), p. 33.

[5]Airola, *How To Get Well,* pp. 214–18; and *How To Keep Slim, Healthy and Young With Juice Fasting* (Phoenix: Health Plus, Publishers, 1974). Herbert M. Shelton, *Fasting Can Save Your Life* (Chicago: Natural Hygiene Press, 1964).

Chapter 3

[1]Shelton, *Fasting Can Save Your Life,* pp. 117–24.

Chapter 4

[1]Wise, *God Knows I Won't Be Fat Again,* p. 136.

[2]Shelton, *Fasting Can Save Your Life,* p. 33.

[3]Ibid.

[4]Eric N. Rogers, *Fasting, The Phenomenon of Self-Denial* (Nashville: Thomas Nelson, 1976), p. 147.

Chapter 5

[1]Jean G. Wade and Helen Kooiman Hosier, *Eating Your Way to Good Health* (Old Tappan, N.J.: Fleming H. Revell, 1977), p. 24.

[2]Ibid., p. 23.

[3]Shelton, *Fasting Can Save Your Life,* p. 140.

[4]Ibid., p. 141.

[5]Ibid., pp. 26–32.

[6]Ann Wigmore, *Be Your Own Doctor* (New York: Hemisphere Press, n.d.), p. 25.

Chapter 6

[1]Arthur Wallis, *God's Chosen Fast* (Fort Washington, Pa.: Christian Literature Crusade, 1968), p. 10.

Chapter 8

[1]*Matthew Henry's Commentary,* vol. 1 (Old Tappan, N.J.: Fleming H. Revell Co., n.d.), p. 24.

[2]Wade and Hosier, *Eating Your Way to Good Health,* p. 9.

[3]Ibid., pp. 80–82.

Chapter 9

[1]Rogers, *Fasting, The Phenomenon of Self-Denial.*

[2]Wallis, *God's Chosen Fast,* p. 8.

[3]Rogers, *Fasting, The Phenomenon of Self-Denial,* p. 50.

[4]David R. Smith, *Fasting, A Neglected Discipline,* (Fort Washington, Pa.: Christian Literature Crusade, 1954), p. 6.

[5]*The New Schaff-Herzog Encyclopedia of Religious Knowledge,* vol. IV, (Grand Rapids: Baker Book House, 1977), p. 283.

[6]J. Hastings, ed., "Fasting," *Encyclopedia of Religion and Ethics.*

[7]Rogers, Fasting, *The Phenomenon of Self-Denial,* p. 44.

[8]Ibid., p. 46.

[9]*Schaff-Herzog Encyclopedia,* p. 283.

[10]Wallis, *God's Chosen Fast,* pp. 34–35.

[11]Ibid., p. 41.

[12]Smith, *Fasting, A Neglected Discipline,* p. 6.

[13]Ibid., p. 6.

[14]*Schaff-Herzog Encyclopedia,* p. 280.

Chapter 10

[1]Arnold Ehret, *Mucusless Diet Healing System* (Beaumont, Calif.: Ehret Literature Publishing Co., 1972), p. 149.

[2]Ibid.

Chapter 12

[1]Bernard Jensen, *World Keys to Health and Long Life* (Escondido, Calif.: Omni Publishers, 1975).